Healthier *without* Wheat

A NEW UNDERSTANDING OF WHEAT ALLERGIES, CELIAC DISEASE, AND NON-CELIAC GLUTEN INTOLERANCE

DR. STEPHEN WANGEN
THE GLUTEN-FREE DOCTOR

AUTHOR OF
The Irritable Bowel Syndrome Solution

www.HealthierWithoutWheat.com

Innate Health Publishing ✦ Seattle, Washington

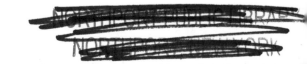

Innate Health Publishing
1229 Madison St, Suite 1220, Seattle, WA, 98104
www.HealthierWithoutWheat.com

Cover design by Kathi Dunn of Dunn+Associates
Book design by Stephanie Martindale

Printed in the USA

10 9 8 7 6 5 4 3 2
    ISBN10 0-9768537-9-5
    ISBN13 978-0-9768537-9-4

Library of Congress Cataloging-in-Publication Data
Wangen, Stephen
    Healthier Without Wheat: A New Understanding
of Wheat Allergies, Celiac Disease, and Non-Celiac Gluten
Intolerance / Stephen Wangen
ISBN 978-0-9768537-9-4
    1. Gluten-Free Diet   2. Celiac Disease   3. Wheat-Free Diet
4. Food Allergies   5. Health

Library of Congress Control Number: 2008925557

The author may be contacted at the IBS Treatment Center:
www.IBSTreatmentCenter.com, info@ibstreatmentcenter.com.

In Remembrance of Louise Shadduck.

1916–2008

Disclaimers

This book is not intended as a substitute for the medical recommendations of physicians or other healthcare providers. It is intended to offer information to help the reader cooperate with physicians and health professionals so that they may work together to find better health.

The publisher and the author are not responsible for any products or services offered or referred to in this book and expressly disclaim all liability in connection with the use of any such products or services and for any damage, loss, or expense to person or property arising out of or relating to them.

All stories contained in this book are based on actual case studies, but the names and other details have been changed.

Dedication

This book is dedicated to the millions of people who suffer from gluten intolerance and lack the support or acknowledgement of the medical community, and the millions more who have yet to be diagnosed with a problem that is sitting on their plate.

It is also dedicated to the numerous researchers who continue to investigate the relationship between food allergies and health, yet rarely get to to see their research put to practical use.

How to contact the IBS Treatment Center

Dr. Wangen and Innate Health Publishing are headquartered at the IBS Treatment Center in Seattle, Washington.

Phone: 206-264-1111
Toll free: 1-888-546-6283, 1-888-5INNATE

Websites:
www.HealthierWithoutWheat.com
www.IBSTreatmentCenter.com

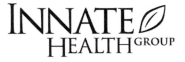

Contents

Acknowledgments

I must thank Marcus Homer Merriman, history professor at the University of Lancaster, England, for once compelling a young student to closely examine the effectiveness of his writing.

This book could not have been written without the help of Susan Fitzgerald, editor extraordinaire. And I wish to thank the Gluten Intolerance Group of North America and its associated branch groups in the Seattle area for giving me voice in my early days as a physician. Largely through their interest and support I developed and refined my knowledge of gluten intolerance.

I would also like to thank my patients, who have had a significant influence on how I practice medicine and have taught me how to provide quality healthcare.

And thank you Tara, Roman, and Lucia for your patience during this long endeavor.

Introduction

When I picture a field of wheat, I can imagine myself enjoying a day of cycling up and down the rolling hills of Middle America. You can probably imagine something similar. Fields of wheat invoke a sense of peace and are almost synonymous with our country, and in a wider sense, wheat is a central part of Western civilization. The importance of this grain to our economy and its assumed presence on our dinner tables might explain our difficulty in perceiving it as a problem. Yet for many, including myself, the grain that is an icon of our culture is also the source of great distress.

This book is about identifying whether or not someone has a problem with wheat or gluten. This is an extremely important subject and may explain why many millions of people suffer from a variety of health concerns. *Healthier Without Wheat* is the result of over 10 years of clinical practice working with and testing thousands of patients. The number of people who react to wheat and gluten, and the profound difference seen in their health when they stop eating them, never ceases to amaze me. This book is also based on a significant amount of independent research published in the medical literature (cited in the bibliography), much of which has focused on celiac disease. That research takes on a whole new meaning when viewed in a different light, a light that I've attempted to brighten with this book.

Things that we take for granted are often not as simple as they appear, and the potential health ramifications of eating wheat is one example of this. Ironically, the public seems to be well ahead of the medical community in appreciating this issue. It is my hope that the medical community will catch up and put itself in a better position to provide answers to the many people who still need our help.

One of the key components to enhancing this educational process can be found in the use of the words *allergy* and *intolerance*. These two words are often used rather loosely or inconsistently, both in the healthcare arena and in the popular vernacular, though they really refer to two very different issues. Because they lack standardization, they often cause confusion when used to discuss reactions to food. I believe that this prevents us from appreciating the true significance of how we react to foods and the full scope of those reactions.

In my first book, *The Irritable Bowel Syndrome Solution*, I attempted to provide a clear foundation for scientifically defining the words *allergy* and *intolerance*. However, when it comes to discussing gluten, I felt that trying to address the differences between them might interfere with the bottom line, which is to help people be healthy. Therefore in this book I have, for the most part, left the debate of allergy versus intolerance alone. However, you will see occasional references to this issue, in particular in the footnotes, which I hope you will find interesting. And I more specifically address it in Chapter 12.

The book is divided into five parts. In Part I, I discuss how wheat became such a major part of our diet and the problems that wheat and gluten cause for many people. In Part II, I discuss celiac disease, which is important to understand in order to appreciate Part III, which examines non-celiac forms of gluten intolerance as well as wheat and gluten allergies. In Part IV, I summarize the information I've presented in earlier chapters on testing for all forms of gluten intolerance and for wheat and gluten allergies. Finally, Part V discusses the treatment of gluten intolerance and, maybe more importantly, what to do when your symptoms aren't relieved by avoiding wheat or gluten, because, although wheat and gluten problems are very important issues, they often go hand in hand with other food allergies and intolerances.

I hope that you find *Healthier Without Wheat* not only informative but thought provoking. And I sincerely hope that it will lead you to a better state of health.

part I

Wheat and the Problems It Can Cause

CHAPTER 1

The Whole of Wheat

Our remedies oft in ourselves do lie.
— William Shakespeare (1564–1616),
All's Well That Ends Well

In a broad sense this is really a story about our assumptions regarding food. We love it. We hate it. We crave it. But do we really understand what we're eating? Almost all of our thoughts about food focus on either satisfying our taste buds or evaluating what it will do to our waistlines. Most people don't consider the most fundamental issue: Did nature ever intend for us to eat what we eat?

Challenging the Health Assumption

Whether or not we are really designed to eat wheat is an incredibly important question. Humans, like all living organisms, are the product of millions of years of evolution. We have been molded by nature to function in a very specific way and when we veer from this design, we suffer consequences. In this way we are not so unlike a car. If you put diesel into a gasoline engine, you wreck the engine. Or consider your favorite zoo animals. Zookeepers try to feed them the same kinds of foods they've been eating for millennia, because they know that the wrong food would make them sick.

However, we humans have a belief that somehow we can overcome or improve upon nature. We eat what we want to eat, or what we are told is good for us, without truly understanding how food and its components affect our bodies.

We make a lot of assumptions about our food. Perhaps the largest is that the major agricultural products in our country are healthy for humans. They may taste good and they may be full of nutrients, but just because something tastes good and contains nutrients doesn't necessarily mean that it is *nutritious*, or nutritious for everyone.

This may sound almost too ridiculous to believe. But as we examine the history of food and the history of humans, you may be surprised to learn that most of what we eat today isn't what humans have eaten throughout most of history. You may also be surprised to learn that what makes up our diet has more to do with economics than with health.

Wheat is part of nearly every meal in America. And most people eat it without a second thought. Yet millions potentially damage their health at nearly every meal without even realizing it. It may be difficult to believe, but it is happening right now and happens every day in numerous households throughout the country. Crazy nonsense, you say? Impossible! How can this be happening?

Food is defined as something that nourishes or sustains us. But what we think of as food, even healthy organic food, isn't necessarily healthy for everyone. We make many assumptions about the health value of the foods that our culture places before us. These assumptions are often surprisingly illogical and are not always supported by sound scientific thought or good medicine. Yet due to a variety of forces, we don't even think to ask the very simplest of questions: "Was I really meant to eat wheat?"

This is a very important question, and the primary question that this book aims to answer. However, in order to address this issue we must challenge conventional thinking. We must consider that something we see every day, something that numerous well-respected and highly educated authorities have told us is very good for us, may not, in fact, be good for a very large number of people.

In order to do this, we have to look at food very differently, and evaluate it for more than just its nutritional content. To help you understand what I mean, consider the well-known parable of the blind men and the elephant from the Buddhist canon:

> It was six men of Indostan
>   To learning much inclined,
> Who went to see the Elephant
>   (Though all of them were blind),
> That each by observation,
>   Might satisfy his mind.
>
> The *First* approached the Elephant,
>   And, happening to fall
> Against his broad and sturdy side,
>   At once began to bawl:
> "God bless me! But the Elephant,
>   Is very like a wall!"
>
> The *Second*, feeling of the tusk,
>   Cried: "Ho! What have we here
> So very round and smooth and sharp?
>   To me 't is mighty clear;
> This wonder of an Elephant,
>   Is very like a spear!"
>
> The *Third* approached the animal,
>   And happening to take
> The squirming trunk within his hands,
>   Thus boldly up and spake:
> "I see," quoth he, "the Elephant
>   Is very like a snake!"

The *Fourth* reached out his eager hand,
  And felt about the knee.
"What most this wondrous beast is like
  Is mighty plain," quoth he;
"'Tis clear enough the Elephant
  Is very like a tree!"

The *Fifth*, who chanced to touch the ear,
  Said; "E'en the blindest man
Can tell what this resembles most;
  Deny the fact who can,
This marvel of an Elephant,
  Is very like a fan!"

The *Sixth* no sooner had begun
  About the beast to grope,
Than, seizing on the swinging tail
  That fell within his scope,
"I see," quoth he, "the Elephant
  Is very like a rope!"

And so these men of Indostan
  Disputed loud and long,
Each in his own opinion
  Exceeding stiff and strong,
Though each was partly in the right,
  And all were in the wrong!

So oft in theologic wars,
  The disputants, I ween,
Rail on in utter ignorance
  Of what each other mean,
And prate about an Elephant,
  Not one of them has seen!

—John Godfrey Saxe (1816–1887)

10

When we look at an issue from only one side, we do not get the whole picture. In our culture, we see wheat as a dietary staple. But for many people we might question whether or not wheat should even be called a food. In some circles a statement like this would be considered not only very strange, but almost unpatriotic. Apparently, this simple grass is more complicated than it first appears.

The History of Wheat

In order to really understand the potential problem with wheat, we need to understand how it has fit into our diet throughout the course of evolution. Until around 10,000 years ago, humans were hunter-gatherers. We hunted game and we gathered what nature provided. Therefore we ate what was in our environment. Depending on the environment and the time of year, this included foods such as fish, wild game, nuts, berries and other fruits, vegetables, leaves, roots, and grass seeds.

Anthropologists know that around 5 million years ago, plant foods made up at least 95% of the human diet, while insects, eggs, and small animals made up the remainder. The fossil record indicates that over time, the amount of harder and more abrasive foods, such as nuts and seeds, and the amount of meat in human diets increased gradually. As humans developed better tools, they were able to hunt larger animals.

It is clear that the human diet was very different than it is today. Grain was not a major source of food for several reasons. Grasses, including the ancestors to wheat, were relatively sparse; they did not grow in vast fields in the same way that we cultivate them today. Second, there was a much larger variety of species available to eat than is typically offered to us now. Third, wild grasses produced very little seed (grain) compared to our modern grasses such as wheat.[1]

Another reason why grain was not commonly eaten is that it is virtually inedible in its raw state. Raw wheat is essentially toxic to humans. Around 10,000 years ago humans discovered that grain can be cooked. The process of cooking the grain broke down most of the toxins and made it edible. Humans also realized that grains can be easily stored and transported, are rich in calories, and produce their own seeds. These realizations aided the development of agriculture.

The wheat we are familiar with in our modern diet is related to a grass that was found in the region of modern-day Syria around 10,000 years ago. Today's wheat has the genetic fingerprint of wild einkorn grass from the Syria-Turkey border area. The cultivation of this grass is thought to have been due to climactic changes occurring around this time as well as to an increase in population, both of which contributed to dwindling and changing food supplies. Rather than leave the food supply up to chance encounters in the environment, people began to grow their own wild grass in order to harvest the seed for food. This was the beginning of the movement away from the hunter-gatherer lifestyle and toward agriculture.

Cereal grains such as wheat provide a large number of calories and can feed a large number of people. Their addition was a major departure from the human diet at any previous point in history. Soon, cultivated grain was a staple food of the region. Einkorn and emmer (two ancestors of wheat), barley, and rye were all

---

1   It is interesting to note that wheat is genetically much more complex than many other living organisms. It has six copies of each gene; most life forms, including humans, have two. Its 21 chromosomes contain 16 billion base pairs of DNA, 40 times as many as rice, 6 times as many as corn, and 5 times as many as people.

grown in this region; all of them contain *gluten*, which we'll discuss later. Wheat, as well as other grains, went from being a very small part of the diet to being an extremely large part of the diet, but only in this region—one in which the people had already had some exposure to this grain. For the humans in other regions of the globe, the ancestors to wheat were not a part of their diet at all. Therefore they had no exposure to the plant that might later dominate the diets of their descendants.

In what is a blink of an evolutionary eye, wheat became a staple of the Middle Eastern and European diets. By 5,000 years ago the cultivation of wheat had reached Ireland, Spain, Ethiopia, and India. By 4,000 years ago it had reached China, long before the cultivation of rice did, although wheat does not play nearly as large a role in the Asian diet as it does in the European or North American diets. Europeans brought it to North America. Although their first attempts at growing grains failed due to the unsuitable Massachusetts soil, they soon enough were able to cultivate the golden fields that are so much a part of our country's image.

The timeline of wheat in the human diet is summarized in Figure 1. Wheat has been bred to have three major beneficial traits that were absent in its wild ancestors: the seeds (grain) are much larger; whole "ears" of grain, rather than individual seeds, grow on each stalk of grass; and the grain is much easier to remove from the stalk, making it easier to harvest. It has been become a plant with numerous extra-large seeds that cannot be dispersed into the wild, dependent entirely on people to reproduce.

Wheat: A Staple in the American Diet

For these reasons we now grow wheat today. It isn't grown because it is the best fuel for our bodies. It is grown because it provides us with an amazing amount of food per acre and is therefore a

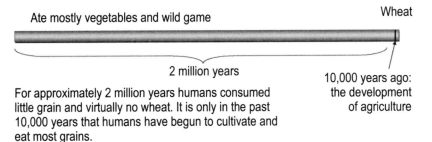

Figure 1. The Natural History of Grain in the Human Diet

very economical food to produce. And people like its taste, which means that it sells. However, many millions of us have not been fortunate enough to inherit the genetic make-up that allows us to enjoy the nutritional benefits of wheat without suffering from one or more of the many potential illnesses that a reaction to wheat can cause.

Wheat is such a mainstay in the American diet that we take it for granted. You might even think that you don't really eat much wheat. But consider this: Without wheat there would be no pasta, no bread (including white bread), no sandwiches, no subs, no bagels, no pretzels, no cookies, no cakes, no Krispy Kremes, no donuts, no pizza, no Raisin Bran, no fish and chips, no Chicken McNuggets, no flour tortillas, no stuffing—the list goes on and on. If you don't recognize the wheat in each of these, don't worry. We'll cover this issue in more detail in Chapter 9.

In North America, a huge amount of the food we eat is made with wheat flour. We eat more wheat per person than any other country. We produce more wheat than any other country. After considering the list above, you might think that it would be impossible to live without eating wheat. This is a common misconception. Most of the foods mentioned above can be made without wheat even though they generally are not.

In fact, entire cultures and billions of people traditionally have had very little, if any, wheat in their diets. This includes those in China, Southeast Asia, Japan, Central America, and South America. They tend to eat much more rice and vegetables than we do. When people from these areas immigrate to the United States, they often have difficulty finding their traditional foods and end up changing their diet into a North American one, and we know that their health suffers. It is also interesting to note that the diet-related health problems so common in the United States are spreading to the Third World as diets there become more like ours.

As our dependence on wheat has grown, we have drastically reduced the amount of fruits and vegetables we eat. This is a cause for concern, even for those whose bodies can tolerate wheat. A major survey of thousands of research studies has concluded that fruits and vegetables have a much higher potential for preventing cancer than do cereal grains. Fruits and vegetables, which used to make up the bulk of the human diet, contain *phytochemicals* that our bodies have grown dependent on over millions of years of evolution. By shifting such a large proportion of our diet from fruits and vegetables to grains, not only have we introduced a new source of potential health problems, we have come to deprive our bodies of what they need to fight disease.

The old saying "You are what you eat" takes on a whole new meaning. If what you eat isn't really meant to be eaten, and if you aren't eating what you *are* meant to eat, then what are you? You're probably not feeling well. You certainly aren't feeling as well as you should. And your body isn't operating at its optimal health.

The Evolution of Health in the United States

Now let's take a brief look at the fundamentals of biology, the science of life. The study of biology is based on the theory of evolution, the principle that nature selects the best-suited organisms to survive and produce offspring. This is a rather subtle process, because it takes place over thousands of years. However, the principle tells us that, as a species, assuming that nothing else has changed, we should be healthier now than we have been at any point in the past.

But things *have* changed. We have antibiotics and immunizations, we have sewage systems and water treatment plants, we produce thousands of doctors and nurses each year to work in hundreds of hospitals, and we spend billions of dollars on healthcare research. Given these positive changes, we as a group should be even healthier than the principle of evolution would predict.

Of course, this is not the way things have turned out. The United States is the most affluent country in the world, spending by far the most money per capita on healthcare, and has an incredibly high-tech healthcare system. Yet, according to the World Health Organization's evaluation of all the nations of the world, the United States ranks 37th in health! How can that be?

In fact, a better question might be this: Is anyone in our country healthy? When you look at the statistics, you might begin to wonder:

+ Approximately 60 million Americans (20%) have irritable bowel syndrome or chronic digestive problems.

+ Approximately 120 million (40%) get heartburn.

+ Between 30 and 60 million (10% to 20%) have severe fatigue.

+ Approximately 15 million (5%, including 10% of all infants) have eczema, 10 million (3%) have dermatitis, and 5.5 million (2%) have psoriasis.

+ Approximately 4 million (1.5%) have fibromyalgia.

+ Approximately 30 million (10%) suffer from depression.

✦ Approximately 45 million (15%) get headaches and 28 million (9%) get migraines.

✦ Approximately 37 million (12%) have arthritis.

✦ Approximately 39 million (13%) suffer from chronic sinusitis.

✦ Approximately 16 million (5%) have diabetes.

✦ Approximately 12 million (4%) have chronic bronchitis.

✦ Approximately 17 million (5.5%) have asthma.

✦ Approximately 61 million (20%) have cardiovascular disease.

✦ And the list goes on and on.

Is this all due to bad genes? If so, how did the genes become bad? Or is it due to our lifestyle? You can't blame all of these problems on being overweight or on a lack of exercise. But, given the startling number of Americans who suffer from one condition or another, it's probably safe to assume that something fundamental to our lives is unhealthy—and in many cases it's something so close to us that we take it for granted.

Summary

Many people know that they have a reaction to wheat or gluten, even though their doctors haven't found any evidence to support the diagnosis. Others may just be beginning to suspect that the symptoms they are experiencing are related to their diets. This book will give both patients and doctors the information they need to understand and appreciate all forms of wheat and gluten intolerance as well as more conventional gluten and wheat allergies.

In this book you will meet a variety of people, like the three described at the end of this chapter, suffering from a wide range of symptoms, from severe digestive problems to skin problems to fatigue and osteoporosis. Some make multiple trips to the emergency room due to extreme pain, while others have no idea that they have a problem. The case studies in the book are compilations of cases seen in clinical practice. Through them you'll learn just how complex reactions to wheat and gluten can be, but you will also see that if you have an intolerance to wheat or gluten, diagnosing and treating it can lead to a marked improvement in your health.

Wheat is not necessarily bad for everyone, and it isn't necessarily the cause of all of the health problems known. However, it is a threat to the good health of the millions of people whose bodies are not able to process it. For these people, as we will see in Chapter 3, the consumption of wheat leads to serious health problems. But first, let's take a closer look at what is inside wheat.

Matthew

Matthew, a 45-year-old engineer, has been experiencing digestive problems for over a year. They started around the time he got an infection but didn't go away when the infection cleared up. On some days he feels okay, but on others he's bloated and his stomach hurts. On the worst days, he has diarrhea.

At first Matthew shrugged off his discomfort, but lately he's found it harder to ignore. He and his wife have always dreamt of traveling, but now that they can finally afford to take a dream vacation, Matthew won't go. He's worried that he would have attacks of diarrhea and the trip would be ruined.

Matthew, who suspects that his symptoms might be tied to his diet, has talked to his doctor several times, but so far he's been unable to find a clear cause. After reading an article about celiac disease, Matthew asked to be tested. His doctor sent him for a blood test, which came back negative. He even went ahead with an endoscopy and a biopsy, but that was negative too. This left Matthew more confused and frustrated than ever.

Laurie

For most of her life, Laurie has been known to her friends and family as a whirlwind of energy, a characteristic that serves her well in her job as a preschool teacher. As a teenager she played several sports and now, at the age of 27, she continues to play soccer in a woman's league.

Several months ago, Laurie started experiencing fatigue. She wasn't just tired—she felt completely worn out. At first she figured she must have picked up a virus from one of her students. But when she felt like her legs were going to give way as she climbed the stairs to her second-floor apartment, she decided to talk to her doctor. Blood tests showed that she has iron deficiency anemia.

Laurie has always been careful about her diet, but now she puts extra effort into making sure that she follows the USDA Food Guide Pyramid, getting all the servings of each food group recommended for a woman her age. She has added iron-rich foods to her diet, including fortified cereals. But she's not feeling any better. In fact, despite her exhaustion she's having trouble sleeping because her legs are so restless that she can't lie still. She is so tired that she's becoming irritable at work and she's missed several weeks of soccer. Her skin is breaking out and last week she was startled to realize that her hair is falling out.

Laurie is now very worried. Her doctor can find no obvious reason for her anemia. No one in her family has it and her periods are not particularly heavy. The changes she's made to her diet don't seem to have helped at all. Her symptoms are affecting her work and her quality of life.

Jim

Although Jim, a 32-year-old, loves to cook and to eat, he's never had trouble with his weight. He gets a lot of exercise, both in his job as a construction worker and with his children, who love to hike, shoot baskets, and swim. His mother and brother have always had sensitive stomachs and have to be careful about what they eat, so Jim has counted himself lucky to be able to eat whatever he wants with few consequences.

Lately, though, Jim has been gaining weight, even though he hasn't changed the way he eats or his activity level. He's also frequently constipated and he sometimes feels sluggish and finds it hard to concentrate. His doctor suggested testing for hypothyroidism, but the results were negative.

Jim's wife, Sarah, wonders if his symptoms could be related to what he's eating. Jim doesn't think so, though, because what he's experiencing is nothing like the cramps and diarrhea that his mother and brother go through when they eat a "problem" food, and he's gaining weight, not losing it. Besides, he's never had trouble with food before.

CHAPTER 2

A Look Inside Wheat: Gluten

It is not the strongest of the species that survive, nor the most intelligent, but the ones most responsive to change.

— Charles Darwin (1809–1882)

The story of unhealthy reactions to wheat is primarily a story about unhealthy reactions to gluten, a *protein* found in wheat. Although other grains, which we will discuss later in this chapter, contain gluten, wheat is the most common source of gluten in most people's diets, and certainly the most attention grabbing. Understanding gluten is imperative to understanding potential problems with wheat. It is also important for understanding why you must avoid so many different grains when you have a gluten intolerance. And it will come in handy later on when we discuss testing for gluten intolerance.

There are over 100 different proteins found in wheat. However, when we talk about an unhealthy reaction to wheat, most of the time we are actually talking about a reaction to gluten. Gluten is really a group of proteins found not only in wheat, but also in several other grains. It is common to use the word *gluten* to represent this group of problematic proteins.

Gluten intolerance is one of the most important health problems in America. It is often mistakenly equated with *celiac disease*. However, celiac disease is really only one form of gluten intolerance. If you are not yet familiar with the terms *gluten intolerance* or *celiac disease*, or if their use seems confusing, consider yourself

21

in good company. We will fully define both of them later, so that by the end of this book you will have a complete understanding of the meaning of each.

Some of the material in this chapter is a bit tricky. If it doesn't make sense right now, don't worry about it. You can skip over those parts for the time being.

Two Different Types of Gluten Intolerance

Gluten intolerance can be divided into two general categories: celiac and non-celiac. Celiac disease is the most recognized form of gluten intolerance and is known to affect about 1% of the population of the United States, which is nearly 3 million people. It can occur at any age and affects people of all ethnic backgrounds. Although the larger medical community readily acknowledges the existence of celiac disease, many doctors still fail to diagnose it because they are not aware of how common this problem is, of the variety of symptoms that it can cause, or of the nearly endless number of combinations of symptoms that can be present or absent in any one person. This happens in spite of the pile of medical research indicating that it is an important and relatively common health problem.

Celiac disease itself is only the tip of the iceberg when it comes to gluten intolerance. As difficult as it sometimes is to find a physician who is well versed in celiac disease and will test for it when it is indicated (which is in a very high number of patients), it is even more difficult to find a doctor who is aware that patients can have a gluten intolerance but not have celiac disease.

In fact, gluten intolerance as a whole is much more common than celiac disease. Although little research has been done on the prevalence of gluten intolerance, it is safe to say, based on clinical experience and a broad public acknowledgement of gluten intolerance, that there are several million people who do not have celiac disease but are gluten intolerant. The percentage of the population that is gluten intolerant is probably close to 10%, which would mean that somewhere in the neighborhood of 30 million Americans suffer from it. And non-celiac gluten intolerance can cause many of the nearly 200 health problems that have been associated with celiac disease. These will be discussed further in the next chapter.

As we've mentioned, the terms *celiac disease* and *gluten intolerance* are usually used interchangeably. This does not accurately reflect the true nature of these conditions. In this book we will establish their differences and fully define each. We will also establish that both conditions are grounded in medical science and can be diagnosed using basic laboratory tests.

When you see the term *gluten intolerance* in this book you may assume that celiac disease is included. However, when you see the word *celiac* you cannot assume that other forms of gluten intolerance are included. In this book the term *celiac disease* will be used only when referring to a very specific type of gluten intolerance.

Gluten Allergies

It is known that some people suffer from what is recognized as a conventional allergic reaction to gluten that is not labeled a gluten intolerance. These people may experience hives; swelling of the lips, tongue, or throat; or other symptoms usually associated with an *allergy*. They are not considered to have a gluten intolerance, but instead are diagnosed as having an *allergy* to gluten. This will be discussed further in Chapter 6. However, through the course of this book we will come to understand that the labels *allergy* and *intolerance* do not always indicate as clear a difference as you might first think.

Wheat Allergies and Intolerances

In addition, a number of people experience reactions to wheat that do not involve gluten and cannot be defined as a gluten intolerance or an allergy to gluten. They react to some part of wheat other than the gluten, and their reaction is limited to wheat and its very close relatives; it does not include most of the other gluten-containing grains. These people are defined as having a *wheat allergy* or *wheat intolerance*. This will be discussed further in Chapter 6.

What Is Gluten?

Gluten is a protein found in many cereal grains and is the main protein in wheat. Gluten is also a type of *prolamin*, a class of simple proteins found in some grains. However, not all prolamins are involved in gluten intolerance and, although you may see this word occasionally, you do not need to be familiar with it to understand gluten.

Gluten is one of the very few things that can make dough elastic and it is vital to the process of making bread. The yeast in the bread recipe ferments the sugars in the grain, creating a gas that is trapped by the dough. The elasticity of gluten allows the dough to stretch and rise, trapping this gas. This is what makes bread light and airy. Without gluten it is difficult to accomplish this feat.

To get a little more technical, there are actually many different subtypes of glutens. Glutens are large carbohydrate-containing proteins, also called *glycoproteins*. While not identical, different types of glutens are very similar. They have similar *amino acid* sequences (which we'll discuss in a moment) and biochemical properties, as well as similar practical properties such as elasticity. They also all seem to have some involvement in gluten intolerance. The singular *gluten* is commonly used when referring to any of these very similar glutens and therefore usually includes the different glutens found in wheat, rye, and barley, as well as in the other gluten-containing grains we'll discuss later.

Note that corn gluten is very different from the gluten referred to in this chapter. Corn gluten is not a problem for people with gluten intolerance, nor is rice gluten.

What Is Gliadin?

Glutens are divided into two broad categories: *gliadins* and glutenins. The gliadins and glutenins involved in gluten intolerance are resistant to digestion by stomach acid and pancreatic enzymes, the two major forms of digestion in your digestive tract. Therefore the digestive process does not break them down into smaller components that can be more easily managed. This may be a primary factor in gluten intolerance.

Gliadins and glutenins both appear to be involved in gluten intolerance, but most research focuses on gliadins, and you may already be familiar with this word. Although there are many different types of gliadins, the singular *gliadin* is usually used when referring to the issue of gliadins in general. Doctors often test for a reaction to gliadin when they are looking for gluten intolerance. This topic will be discussed in detail in the chapters on celiac disease and non-celiac gluten intolerance.

Gliadins are rich in *glutamine* and *proline*, two important amino acids. Amino acids are essential to life and when linked together form proteins. To give you an idea about how large gliadins are, one of the glutamine-rich gliadins that is particularly problematic in gluten intolerance has 33 amino acids. Do not be confused by the fact that gliadins contain glutamine. This does not mean that glutamine is a problem for people who are gluten intolerant, nor does it mean that glutamine should be avoided. In fact, just the opposite is true and we will discuss this in the chapter on treating gluten intolerance.

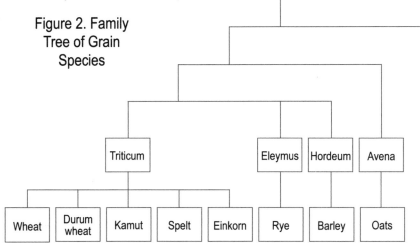

Notice that the grasses in the Triticum grouping are very closely related. They are each high in gluten. Rye and barley also contain gluten. None of the other grasses shown here contain gluten, and you can see that they become more distantly related to wheat as you move from left to right.

Figure 2. Family Tree of Grain Species

Where Is Gluten?

If you're thinking, "Enough with the technical stuff. Just tell me which foods contain gluten," that is understandable. As mentioned earlier, wheat is the most common source of gluten in most people's diets. However, many other plants that we eat contain gluten.

Consider the family tree of grain species shown in Figure 2. The grains that belong to the triticum grouping—wheat, durum wheat, kamut, spelt, and einkorn—are high in gluten. Rye and barley, which are closely related to the triticum grasses, also contain gluten. The grains to the right of these do not contain this problematic gluten. We can see that the more closely related a grain is to wheat, the more similar is its gluten content and the more likely it is to be a problem for those suffering from gluten intolerance.

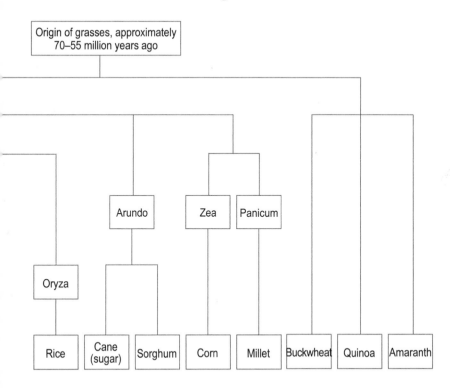

Gluten is found in the following grains, and subsequently in just about everything made from them:

- Wheat
- Spelt
- Rye
- Barley
- Kamut
- Durum
- Triticale
- Einkorn
- Semolina
- Bulgur
- Wheat germ
- Couscous
- Farina
- Emmer
- Matzoh
- Graham

For more information about the many processed foods that contain these grains, please see Chapter 9 and refer to the excellent books listed in Appendix B.

There is a great deal of confusion and misinformation about which grains contain gluten. Therefore, it should be clarified that the following grains do *not* contain gluten:

- Amaranth
- Millet
- Sorghum
- Buckwheat
- Oats[2]
- Teff
- Corn
- Rice

Many of the books referred to in Appendix B also discuss foods that are gluten free and safe to eat for people who are gluten intolerant.

Joe

Food was one of the pleasures of Joe's life. Grateful that he didn't suffer from the digestive problems that his siblings have, Joseph long ago decided that he wouldn't watch every bite that went into his mouth. Between his job as a high school PE teacher and his family life he got plenty of exercise, so he felt that — within moderation — he should be able to eat what he wanted.

During the week, Joe started his day with a quick breakfast — a bowl of cereal or toast and fruit. On the weekends, he and his children made a big breakfast together; the kids' favorites were blueberry pancakes and French toast. Joe usually brought a sandwich to work for lunch, but sometimes he would grab a hotdog or hamburger from the school cafeteria.

To Joe, the best time of day is dinnertime. He and his wife, Lisa, share a love of cooking and usually make dinner together. Nothing is more relaxing than spending this time with his family, catching up on the day's news. On most days, they ate a traditional sit-down dinner together, which

---

2 Although note that oats are often contaminated with gluten; see "About Oats" later in this chapter.

always included fresh bread or rolls. On evenings when the kids had a practice, they might grab a fast-food meal. Once every couple of weeks, Joe and Lisa treated themselves to dinner at a local Italian or Mexican restaurant.

Joe didn't drink a lot of alcohol, but he did enjoy his beer. He sometimes went out after work on Fridays, and weekends often included time spent watching sports with a beer and a big bowl of tortilla chips.

Overall, Joe's diet was a pretty typical one for a family guy. Not everything he ate was healthy, but, because he stuck to his motto — "Everything in moderation" — he never had to worry about his weight. That is until several months ago, when he started steadily gaining weight. He also began suffering from cramps after he ate. At first he didn't relate the two symptoms, thinking the cramps might be caused by a bug, but when they didn't go away, he began to wonder if his carefree eating days were over.

After consulting his doctor, who, being celiac himself, was very familiar with food intolerances, Joe underwent testing and was diagnosed with a gluten intolerance. Until he was faced with adopting a gluten-free diet, he had never thought about just how much gluten he ingested every day, from his breakfast to his after-work beer. Changing the way he eats has been a big challenge, but he's found a lot of alternative products which are safe for him. He's realized that he has a choice: he can eat the way he used to and jeopardize his health, or he can adapt to this new way of eating and keep his active lifestyle. To him, the decision was easy.

About Oats

There has been a great deal of debate over the years about whether or not oats are a problem for people with a gluten intolerance. Studies have established that oats do not in fact contain gluten or gliadin of the type contained in wheat, barley, rye, and so on. However, oats almost always get contaminated with other grains. This can happen in the field; during harvesting, transportation, and storage; or during processing.

Therefore it is recommended that people diagnosed with a gluten intolerance, including celiac disease, or who are otherwise very sensitive to gluten should avoid oats. That being said, some companies now produce truly gluten-free oats. They take great care to keep all oats strictly separate from other grains at every stage, from cultivation to processing. Oats from these companies are fine for people with a gluten intolerance. They are listed in Appendix C.

Keep in mind that it is possible to be reactive to oats, independent of whether or not you have a reaction to gluten. This can be tested for, but it is not a common practice to do so. If you notice a reaction to oats, it may be that you are intolerant of oats as well as gluten.

Brenda

Just before her 45th birthday, Brenda was in an accident. Soon after, she began experiencing migraines. Like many people, she'd had many headaches in her life, but never ones like these. If one came on at work, she had to call her husband to pick her up because she couldn't even drive home. Brenda did some reading on migraines and felt that they were probably caused by the onset of menopause.

Over the next few months, however, she started suffering from stomach cramps and bouts of diarrhea. "I'm falling apart as I'm getting older," she joked with her family.

When her digestive problems started interfering with her everyday life, she consulted her doctor. After a series of tests, she was diagnosed with a gluten intolerance. Her doctor told her that this could be causing her headaches as well and advised her to stop eating wheat.

When Brenda eliminated all wheat from her diet, her symptoms improved, but they didn't go away as she'd expected them to. Her friend Sara, who used to suffer from IBS, suggested that Brenda consult another doctor, who had helped Sara discover which foods caused problems for her. Brenda learned from this doctor that other grains — including some she was eating instead of wheat — contain gluten. The doctor also told her that oats can be contaminated with gluten-containing grains.

Brenda has changed her diet again, eliminating all grains with gluten and switching to a different brand of oats. She's been pleased to discover that there are still many grains that are safe for her to eat. Now she's on a truly gluten-free diet and the migraines and digestive problems have resolved and no longer interfere with her day.

Summary

Gluten is a protein found in wheat, barley, rye, and several other grains. While types of gluten are also found in other plants in our diet, such as corn and rice, only those types found in the close wheat relatives play a role in gluten intolerance.

As mentioned, there are many different forms of gluten intolerance, including the most widely known, celiac disease, as well as non-celiac gluten intolerance. Less commonly seen are other types of wheat allergies that do not necessarily involve gluten, as well as a conventional gluten allergy, which is distinct from what is usually referred to as a gluten intolerance. Each of these topics will be covered in more detail later in this book.

With this basic understanding of what gluten is and where it is found, we can move on to the types of problems it can cause.

CHAPTER 3

Reacting to Wheat: The Many Faces of Gluten Intolerance and Gluten-Associated Diseases

What is food to one may be fierce poison to others.
— Lucretius (c. 99 B.C.–c. 55 B.C.),
Roman Epicurean poet, philosopher, and scientist

Gluten intolerance can cause a surprisingly wide variety of symptoms[3] and health problems. While most people associate gluten intolerance with digestive problems, it can also cause or is associated with[4] complications far beyond the digestive tract. It has been well established that a gluten intolerance can dramatically affect the skin, nervous system, musculoskeletal system, immune system, energy level, joints, teeth, and even behavior and mood.

---

3   In the medical community, a distinction is made between *signs* and *symptoms*. A sign is objective and observable by someone other than the patient; for example a rash, or a test result showing low iron stores, are both signs. A symptom, in contrast, is subjective, and cannot be directly observed; for example, abdominal pain is a symptom. For the purposes of this book, however, we use *symptom* for both of these in order to avoid complicating the discussion.

4   To say that gluten intolerance *causes* a problem means that we know that the gluten intolerance is responsible for the symptom or damage. To say that it is *associated with* or *correlated with* the problem means that we often see the symptom or damage in people who are gluten intolerant, but we aren't sure if the gluten intolerance is the actual cause of it. That is, we know only that the two issues tend to co-occur. It may be a causal relationship, but we haven't proven it yet.

The conditions associated with gluten intolerance are so varied that after reading the complete list presented in this chapter, you might think that everyone has a gluten intolerance. Of course, this is not the case, but several million people in the United States are gluten intolerant and are completely unaware of it. It is very important to understand that just because someone has a gluten intolerance, this does not guarantee that he or she will have a particular problem or symptom. Nor will he or she have all of the conditions listed in this chapter. In fact, some people who notice no symptoms whatsoever still test positive for and have a gluten intolerance.

It is also important to understand that there are many possible causes for most of the problems discussed in this chapter. This is because these problems are really just signs or symptoms of some deeper issue. For example, fatigue has numerous possible causes, including iron deficiency, insomnia, stress, hypothyroidism, staying up too late, and poor diet, to name just a few. Having fatigue does not automatically mean that you have a gluten intolerance.

Having said this, two specific reactions are generally considered to be caused only by a gluten intolerance. These are *villous atrophy* of the small intestine[5] and *dermatitis herpetiformis*, and they will be discussed in much more detail in the next chapter. If you don't know what they are or can't even pronounce them, read on anyway.

It's Not Just a Digestive Problem

As mentioned above, a reaction to gluten can lead to many health issues. Traditionally, gluten intolerance was thought to cause only digestive problems, including diarrhea, weight loss, abdominal pain, gas, and bloating. More recently, researchers and physicians

---

5   However, some research indicates that villous atrophy can be caused by conditions other than gluten intolerance. This will be discussed in the next chapter.

have come to realize that only a small percentage of people who are gluten intolerant have these problems. Research, as well as feedback from patients, has shown that a tremendous number of problems can be triggered by a gluten intolerance. Many people actually have symptoms completely opposite of those that we used to think defined a gluten intolerance — they suffer from constipation and weight gain triggered by gluten. In fact, many celiacs are overweight when they are diagnosed with celiac disease.

Other gluten intolerant people suffer from one or more of a wide variety of health problems. In this chapter, we will discuss these problems and attempt to explain why so many different health issues can be caused by a reaction to gluten. Because there are so many, it is helpful to break them down into categories. And rather than introduce them all at once, we will begin with some of the more common problems, as the complete list is a bit overwhelming and many of the conditions included in it are relatively uncommon. First, let's consider some differences between infants and toddlers on one hand and adults and older children on the other.

Problems Commonly Seen in Infants and Toddlers

Infants and toddlers suffering from a gluten intolerance tend to experience certain problems more commonly than older children and adults. However, symptoms can show up at any age, and we should re-emphasize that just because an infant or toddler doesn't have any health problems, it doesn't mean that they don't have a gluten intolerance which will cause them problems later in life. Some of the more common problems caused by a gluten intolerance in infants and toddlers include the following:

✦ Colic
✦ Fatigue
✦ Diarrhea

✦ Gas
✦ Vomiting
✦ Projectile vomiting
✦ Failure to thrive/poor growth
✦ Refusal to eat
✦ Bloated abdomen
✦ Eczema
✦ Constipation
✦ Poor sleep
✦ Angry disposition
✦ Chronic ear infections

As mentioned above, there are many possible reasons for which an infant or toddler can have these symptoms. If your child has any of these problems, it is important to find out the underlying cause and not just treat the symptom. Medications that only suppress symptoms may provide immediate relief, but they can mask a much larger issue and prevent you from diagnosing a problem that could have long-term effects on the health of your child. Infants and children are discussed in more detail in Chapter 8.

Problems Commonly Seen in Adults and Older Children
As we've stated, the variety of conditions associated with gluten intolerance is enormous. However, with adults and children, as with infants and toddlers, some are much more common than others. Here is the short list of problems most commonly seen in gluten intolerance:

✦ Diarrhea
✦ Constipation
✦ Heartburn
✦ Abdominal pain

✦ Headaches (including migraines)
✦ Fatigue
✦ Muscle aches
✦ Joint pain
✦ Hypoglycemia
✦ Eczema
✦ Acne
✦ Mental fogginess
✦ Anemia (iron or B12 deficiency)
✦ Frequent illness
✦ Itchy skin
✦ Low bone density

The Complete List

These are short lists above. But the following pages present a complete list of the nearly 200 problems associated with gluten intolerance, sorted into 13 categories: digestive, skin, emotional, physical well-being, mind/neurological, musculoskeletal, respiratory, head, women's health, autoimmune, chromosomal defects, malignancies/cancer, and miscellaneous. In some cases a problem clearly falls into more than one category and is listed in both.[6] Remember, a gluten-intolerant person may have none, one, or several of these symptoms or conditions. Although most of these problems can have other causes, a gluten intolerance can be associated with any of them and is known to cause many of them.

✦ **Digestive**
Abdominal pain
Aphthous ulcers
Autoimmune hepatitis

---

6   An alphabetical listing of these symptoms can be found in the appendix.

Bloating

Canker sores

Colon cancer

Constipation

Cramping

Diarrhea

Dyspepsia

Elevated liver enzymes (ALT, ALK, ALP)

Elevated transaminases

Enamel defects in teeth

Encopresis

Eosinophilic esophagitis

Eosinophilic gastroenteritis

Esophagitis

Fructose intolerance

Gas

Gastroesophageal reflux disease (GERD)

Gastroparesis

Heartburn

Hepatic steatosis

Hepatic T-cell lymphoma

Intestinal bleeding

Irritable bowel syndrome (IBS)

Lactose intolerance

Liver disease

Nausea

Occult blood in stool

Impaired pancreatic exocrine function

Pancreatitis

Primary biliary cirrhosis

Primary sclerosing cholangitis

Reflux

Sore throat, chronic

Steatorrhea (fatty stools)

Villous atrophy

Vomiting

✦ **Skin**

Acne

Eczema

Dermatitis

Dermatitis herpetiformis

Dry skin

Follicular keratosis

Hives

Rashes

Itchiness

Psoriasis welts

Redness

Dark circles under eyes

Linear IgA bullous dermatosis

Urticaria

Hereditary angioneurotic edema

Cutaneous vasculitis

Erythema nodosum

Erythema elevatum diutinum

Necrolytic migratory erythema

Vitiligo disease

Behçet's disease

Oral lichen planus

Dermatomyositis

Porphyria

Alopecia areata (hair loss)

Acquired hypertrichosis lanuginosa
Pyoderma gangrenosum
Ichthyosiform dermatoses
Pellagra
Generalized acquired cutis laxa
Atypical mole syndrome and congenital giant nevus

✦ **Emotional**
Anxiety
Irritability
Depression
Ups and downs

✦ **Physical well-being**
Fatigue
Weight loss
Weight gain
Poor endurance
Inability to gain weight
Chronic fatigue
Failure to thrive
Short stature

✦ **Mind/Neurological**
Autism
Attention deficit hyperactivity disorder (ADHD)
Difficulty concentrating
Cerebellar atrophy
Mental fog
Brain white-matter lesions
Insomnia/difficulty sleeping
Schizophrenia
Ataxia/difficulty with balance

Epilepsy
Multifocal axonal polyneuropathy
Peripheral neuropathy (numbness or tingling of hands or feet)
Rett Syndrome

✦ **Musculoskeletal**
Arthritis
Fibromyalgia
Rheumatoid arthritis
Muscle aches
Joint pain
Osteoporosis
Osteopenia
Osteomalacia
Polymyositis
Loss of strength
Short stature
Multiple sclerosis
Myasthenia gravis

✦ **Respiratory**
Wheezing
Chronic sinusitis
Shortness of breath
Asthma

✦ **Women's health**
Irregular cycle
Infertility (also male infertility)
Delayed start of menstruation
Premature menopause
Spontaneous abortion/miscarriage

✦ **Head**
Headaches
Migraines
Alopecia areata (hair loss)

✦ **Chromosomal defects**
Down Syndrome

✦ **Miscellaneous**
Anemia
Iron deficiency
Vitamin B12 deficiency (pernicious anemia)
Vitamin K deficiency
Folate deficiency
Impotency
Raynaud's
Elevated eosinophils in blood test
Cystic fibrosis
Pulmonary hemosiderosis

✦ **Autoimmune disorders**
Addison's disease
Autoimmune chronic hepatitis
Alopecia areata (hair loss)
Type 1 diabetes
Graves' disease
Secondary hyperparathyroidism
Hypothyroidism, autoimmune
Idiopathic autoimmune hypoparathyroidism
Idiopathic thrombocytopenic purpura (ITP)
Lupus (SLE)

Myasthenia gravis
Sarcoidosis
Scleroderma
Sjogrens syndrome
Thyroiditis
Villous atrophy

✦ **Malignancies/Cancer**
Colon cancer
Esophageal and oro-pharyngeal carcinoma
Melanoma
Non-Hodgkin's lymphoma
Small bowel adenocarcinoma

As you can see, gluten intolerance is associated with just about
every part of your body. You might think that the number of conditions associated with it is unbelievably long. However, asso-
ciations between most of these conditions and gluten intolerance
are substantiated in the medical literature (an extensive reference
list is provided in the bibliography). Links with the others have
been seen in clinical practice. Most of the research done so far has
focused on the relationship between these conditions and celiac
disease rather than on the broader issue of gluten intolerance.
This leaves open the possibility that there may be other conditions
associated with gluten intolerance.

Angela

Angela, a recently retired bank manager, considered herself
relatively healthy throughout her life. She did have a history
of chronic ear infections as a child and as an adult she's had
to deal with eczema, but she has had no serious illnesses.
As she's gotten older, Angela has noticed that she's not as

mentally sharp as she used to be, but until recently she attributed this to the normal effects of aging.

When Angela turned 65, her doctor recommended that she have a routine bone density scan. Angela had no risk factors for osteoporosis — her weight is in the normal range, she has no family history of bone problems, and she's never smoked. In fact, ever since she read an article on preventing osteoporosis many years ago, she has faithfully taken a daily calcium supplement, made sure that her diet includes a variety of dairy products, and exercised regularly. So the results of the scan came as a big surprise.

"Why would I have low bone density?" she asked her doctor. While her doctor assured her that the diagnosis was not out of the ordinary for someone her age, Angela wanted to find out if that was the whole story.

So Angela did some reading to try to figure out why, despite her efforts, she had developed this condition. She learned that some underlying conditions can keep your body from absorbing nutrients, including calcium, so she asked her doctor to have her tested for them. The test for gluten intolerance came back positive.

Angela, who feels that it's important to take responsibility for your own healthcare, undertook more research, this time to learn as much about gluten intolerance as she could. She discovered that the seemingly unrelated health issues she's had in her life can all be associated with gluten intolerance.

"Now that I'm on a gluten-free diet, my skin is much better," she told her doctor, "and I feel much more 'with it.' It's such a relief to know that my fogginess wasn't irreversible or due to aging." Angela feels fortunate that her intolerance was discovered before she developed more serious health problems.

Why So Many Problems?

By now you might be asking, "How can such a mixed bag of problems be associated with gluten intolerance?" That is a good question. Most of the symptoms and conditions listed above can be separated into two broad classifications: those caused by the *malabsorption* of nutrients and those caused by an immune reaction, most notably *inflammation*.

Malabsorption

We often assume that what we eat is automatically absorbed and utilized by the body. However, for one reason or another, your body may not absorb all the nutrients from your food. An obvious cause of malabsorption is diarrhea, in which nutrients pass right through the body before they have much chance to be absorbed. But malabsorption can also occur when there is no diarrhea.

A gluten intolerance is a reaction to gluten that begins in the digestive tract. This logically leads to poor digestion and less than optimal absorption of nutrients from any foods that contain gluten and from many of the other foods eaten in conjunction with gluten. Conditions directly related to the malabsorption of nutrients include the following:

- ✦ Fatigue
- ✦ Failure to thrive/poor growth
- ✦ Enamel defects in teeth
- ✦ Hypoglycemia
- ✦ Iron deficiency anemia
- ✦ Loss of strength
- ✦ Vitamin B12 deficiency anemia
- ✦ Pernicious anemia
- ✦ Osteomalacia
- ✦ Osteopenia

+ Osteoporosis
+ Weight loss
+ Poor endurance
+ Inability to gain weight

Reduced bone density, whether in the form of osteoporosis or osteopenia, is relatively common in both adults and children with celiac disease, especially in those with diarrhea. This, of course, increases their risk for fractures. Bone density generally increases once these people start following a gluten-free diet. However, if you are in your 20s or older, have celiac disease, and have suffered from diarrhea, it is a good idea to undergo a bone density scan. It is better to know about this problem earlier rather than later.

These are the most obvious conditions related to the malabsorption of nutrients. Others, such as migraines and depression, may be caused by nutritional deficiencies due to malabsorption or by a combination of malabsorption and inflammation. The research on nutrients and their relationship to conditions such as these is far too extensive to go into here.

Inflammation

Inflammation is a direct result of the immune system being activated to do its job. Because in gluten intolerance the immune system reacts to food, it has the potential to set off a wide range of inflammatory conditions throughout the body. Most of the conditions on the master list can be traced back to the immune system and the inflammatory response, including nearly all of the skin conditions, most of the digestive problems, and all of the autoimmune conditions.[7] Many of the other conditions listed are also directly related to the immune response and inflammation.

---

7   The author proposes that we may eventually link cardiovascular diseases and other inflammatory-based disorders such as Alzheimer's and Parkinson's to immune reactions to food.

Other Specific Issues

A few areas deserve special attention because more research has
been done on them and we know a little more about their relationship with gluten intolerance. These conditions can still be
classified as being related to the immune response, nutritional
deficiencies, or both.

✦ Malignancies/Cancer

Three types of cancer in particular occur more commonly in
people with celiac disease. These are small bowel adenocarcinoma,
espohageal and oro-pharyngeal squamous cell carcinoma, and
non-Hodgkin's lymphoma. Celiac disease is not the only condition related to these cancers, but it does increase the likelihood
that they will occur.

Most research supports the belief that a gluten-free diet can
protect those with celiac disease against the development of
these cancers. For example, the risk for developing small bowel
adenocarcinoma is 80 times higher in untreated celiacs than in the
general population. This risk appears to be reduced dramatically
once a gluten-free diet has been implemented. However, one study
has suggested that the risk of non-Hodgkin's lymphoma may
remain higher for those with celiac disease in spite of a gluten-
free diet.

These risk factors emphasize the need for regular physical exams
and, at a minimum, keeping up with age-appropriate occult blood
testing (measuring blood in the stool, possible causes of which
include polyps or cancer, among others) and colonoscopies
(visually examining the colon for abnormalities).

✦ Eosinophils

Eosinophils are a type of white blood cell. They can be measured
on a routine complete blood count (CBC). Or, a tissue sample,

such as a biopsy, may reveal abnormally high levels of them. People with gluten intolerance sometimes have elevated eosinophils in the blood or have conditions such as eosinophilic esophagitis or eosinophilic gastroenteritis. If you have any type of elevated eosinophils, be sure to be screened for gluten intolerance.

✦ Fertility

Celiac disease is known to affect female fertility in a variety of ways, including delaying the age of onset of menstruation and contributing to amenorrhea (lack of menstruation), recurrent spontaneous abortions (miscarriages), and premature menopause. Celiac disease is also known to affect male fertility. In addition, it may lead to low birth-weight babies or a shorter than normal time for breast-feeding. Some studies have shown that a gluten-free diet improves these issues and, in some cases, can completely resolve them.

✦ Autoimmune Disorders

The purpose of the immune system is to attack foreign invaders, such as bacteria, viruses, or even food. But in those with an *autoimmune disorder*, the immune system attacks part of the body itself. Celiac disease is an autoimmune condition; this will be discussed in the next chapter. Other autoimmune disorders occur 10 times more often in those with celiac disease than in the general population.

We don't know exactly why those with celiac disease are more prone to autoimmune disorders. But it is possible that autoimmune diseases can be prevented in celiacs who are diagnosed early and follow a gluten-free diet. If the autoimmune disease is already present, it may improve on a gluten-free diet, but this does not appear to be common.

✦ Neurological Problems

A number of neurological problems are associated with gluten intolerance. These range from schizophrenia to epilepsy to simple brain fog. Interestingly, there are several medical articles published on these issues and their relationship to gluten intolerance. There has also been an excellent book written on this subject by Dr. Rodney Ford titled *Full of It*. These problems may or may not be related to the immune reaction to gluten or the malabsorption of nutrients. But there can be no doubt that gluten intolerance can have a profound effect on one's mental health.

Why Do Different People Get Different Symptoms?

Why does gluten intolerance seem to exhibit itself so differently in different people? This is the $6 million question. No one really knows the answer, but it is most likely related to genetics and various other influences on our health.

As we've seen, there is no simple one-to-one relationship between gluten and the problems that it causes. And this is probably the biggest obstacle to getting doctors to test for celiac disease or gluten intolerance. Doctors generally expect things to be much more straightforward than this; they are used to something much closer to one cause for each problem and one treatment for each problem. Gluten intolerance definitely doesn't fit this model.

Can Gluten Be Addictive?

Nearly 30 years ago researchers discovered a fact that has now been well established, that gluten contains peptide chemicals that act as *opioids*, meaning they have an opiate-like effect. Other foods, including dairy, rice, beef, and even spinach, are also known to contain some amount of opioids.

Opiates act on the neurological system by enhancing the effects of neurotransmitters known as endorphins. They suppress pain, reduce anxiety, and, at sufficiently high doses, produce euphoria. Opiates are natural compounds, but are also used as narcotics to treat a variety of problems, most commonly pain (examples of opiate pain medications include hydrocodone [Vicodin], oxycodone [Percodan, OxyContin], and meperidine [Demerol]); cough (codeine); and diarrhea (loperamide), and to help people addicted to heroin (methadone). Many of these drugs are habit forming and have a variety of potential side effects.

It is interesting to note that many patients express that they feel almost as if they are addicted to gluten, and people often find it very difficult to give up. Those who know that gluten contains opioids hypothesize that this is the reason why. An entire movement has based its avoidance of gluten (and, in some cases, dairy) on this previously little-known fact, popularized by the book *Dangerous Grains* by Dr. James Braly and Ron Hoggan. Very little research has been done on the impact of the opioids in food on humans. The few studies that have been done have focused on animals. If the opioid activity of these foods is significant, it very likely affects different people in different ways, as do opiates.

Many parents of autistic children have long believed that avoiding gluten and dairy provides significant benefits to their children. And the medical literature contains hypotheses that there is a correlation between schizophrenia and the ingestion of gluten. While much more research is needed, the opiate-like activity of gluten is certainly interesting in light of the many psychological, emotional, mental, and behavioral problems associated with gluten intolerance.

It should be pointed out that there is no known relationship between gluten intolerance and the fact that gluten contains opioids.

However, if a gluten intolerance leads to intestinal damage that makes the lining of the digestive tract more permeable, as it does in those with celiac disease, it is possible that more opioids are absorbed. This could potentially lead to an increase in the opiate-like effects of gluten.

Summary

In this chapter we've seen that gluten intolerance causes or is associated with a wide variety of health conditions, most of which are related to the effects of malabsorption or inflammation. A gluten-intolerant person may have one, some, or none of these problems, and this lack of consistency makes it difficult for doctors to recognize that testing for gluten intolerance is called for.

part II

Celiac Disease

CHAPTER 4

Understanding and Testing for Celiac Disease

What is wanted is not the will to believe, but the wish to find out, which is the exact opposite.
—Bertrand Russell (1872–1970), Sceptical Essays, 1928

Whether or not you have celiac disease, you should read this chapter. In order to understand the various forms of gluten intolerance, we first need to define celiac disease. This will make it much easier to understand why celiac disease is not the same thing as gluten intolerance. It is a very specific type of gluten intolerance that does not represent the multitude of forms of gluten intolerance.

This chapter also describes the various methods for testing for celiac disease and their relative merit. Understanding these tests helps put celiac disease into its proper place within the larger arena of gluten intolerance. However, if you find some parts too technical or just plain boring, then skip over them. You may find that you later want to come back to this chapter to gather a few more details on celiac disease. Other forms of gluten intolerance and the methods for testing for them are explored in the next chapter.

What Happens to the Body in Celiac Disease?

In people with celiac disease, eating gluten leads to a very specific type of damage to the *villi* in the small intestine. Villi are finger-like extensions of the surface of the intestinal tract, so small that they can be seen only under a microscope. Although they are tiny, your villi are important to your health because together they make up a very large portion of the surface area of your small intestine.

In people with celiac disease, the villi are worn down or blunted. This is known as *villous atrophy*. It is something like the difference between holding your hand open with your fingers out and having your hand clenched into a fist. Your extended fingers are like healthy villi. The knuckles on your fist represent the blunted villi. You can see that when your fingers are extended, the surface area of your hand is larger than when they are curled. If your villi are blunted, then the surface area of your small intestine is much smaller than it should be. This in turn means that your body cannot absorb nutrients very well, which can lead to the variety of conditions caused by malabsorption that were listed in the previous chapter.

The most important thing to know about all of this is that celiac disease is defined by villous atrophy. If you do not have villous atrophy, then you do not have celiac disease.[8]

How Do Villi Get Damaged?

When someone with celiac disease eats gluten, his or her immune system is triggered to attack not only the gluten, but also his or her own intestinal tract. We do not know exactly why this happens, but it appears to be a genetic response to gluten. This is an auto-immune reaction because the immune system is attacking part of the body. Thus, celiac disease is an autoimmune disorder.

The attack against the villi is an attack against the endomysium, the lining of the small intestine. The specific part of the endomysium that is being attacked is an *enzyme* known as *tissue transglutaminase*. It is the job of this enzyme to repair damage to

---

8   Note that villous atrophy is included in the list of symptoms and conditions related to gluten intolerance provided in the previous chapter, under both digestive disorders and autoimmune diseases. We could have used the term *celiac disease* in place of *villous atrophy* on that list.

the lining of the small intestine. But when the enzyme is attacked, it cannot do its job. This, of course, results in damage to the small intestine, which leads to villous atrophy.

Other Names for Celiac Disease

Celiac disease can be referred to by many different names, depending on the habits of your healthcare provider and the country that you are in. You may see or hear the following terms used in reference to celiac disease:

- ✦ Celiac sprue
- ✦ Celiacs
- ✦ Coeliac disease
- ✦ Gee-Herter's syndrome
- ✦ Gluten intolerance
- ✦ Gluten sensitive enteropathy
- ✦ Gluten sensitivity
- ✦ Non-tropical sprue

Whether or not these names—in particular *gluten intolerance* and *gluten sensitivity*—should be used interchangeably with *celiac disease* is an important issue and will be discussed in the next chapter.

Who Gets Celiac Disease?

While traditionally not widely known, celiac disease is actually a fairly common problem. In fact, studies show that nearly 3 million people in the United States—at least 1 out of every 133—have it. It can be found in people of all ages, including very young children, but only after gluten has been introduced to the diet. It also does not discriminate between men and women. Although it is really more of an allergy than a disease, it is typically called a gluten intolerance rather than a gluten allergy.[9]

For a long time it was thought that only people of northern European descent got celiac disease. However, this belief was based on incomplete information. As often happens, you don't find what you aren't looking for. Once people from other parts of the world were studied, it became clear that celiac disease is not just a European or North American issue. And why would it be? There is no logical reason to think that people in other parts of the world would be any more tolerant of gluten than Caucasians.

Celiac disease has been found to be just about as prevalent in Turkey, Iran, Iraq, Saudi Arabia, Jordan, and Kuwait as it is in the United States. It has also been found in Egypt, Tunisia, Algeria, and Libya, as well as Brazil, Argentina, Venezuela, Uruguay, Chile, Mexico, and Cuba. And let's not leave out Australia and New Zealand. India? Yes. Japan and China? Yes. The rest of the world? Who knows? We haven't checked there yet.

What Are the Symptoms of Celiac Disease?

As with all gluten intolerances, the symptoms of celiac disease vary widely. Celiac disease is typically thought of as causing diarrhea, abdominal pain, gas, and bloating. However, recent studies have

---

9   I prefer to call these *allergies*, because an allergy is a reaction caused by an immune response. Celiac disease and most forms of gluten intolerance involve an immune system reaction to gluten. I believe that using the word *allergy* is far more accurate than using *intolerance*, as I established in my book *The Irritable Bowel Syndrome Solution*. As an example, a gluten intolerance and a lactose intolerance are two completely different issues that have nothing in common. A lactose intolerance is an enzyme deficiency and does not involve the immune system. However, it is common to use the phrase *gluten intolerance* when referring to an immune reaction to gluten. Although I consider this an inaccurate use of *intolerance*, I feel that the most important issue in this book is to recognize that there are many ways of reacting to gluten. Therefore I have chosen to stick with the common usage of *gluten intolerance*.

clearly shown that most people with celiac disease do not have these symptoms. They may experience experience many other symptoms, including constipation, weight gain, fatigue, headaches, heartburn, skin problems such as eczema and acne, or any number of other health problems discussed in the previous chapter.

It is also not uncommon to have celiac disease and yet not experience any symptoms at all. Recent research indicates that as many as half of those with celiac disease are considered asymptomatic. And a significant percentage of people with celiac disease do not get diagnosed until, after decades of good health, one of the symptoms or problems associated with celiac disease listed in the previous chapter is finally found, such as osteoporosis. Or they may suffer for decades from something such as chronic anemia (iron or B12 deficiency) before they are finally tested for celiac disease.

Testing for Celiac Disease

Celiac disease is diagnosed by evaluating patients for villous atrophy. This can be done in a variety of ways, including an intestinal biopsy and several blood tests. In this section, we'll discuss each of them, as well as genetic testing, in detail.

Positive Versus Negative Test Results

So that there isn't any confusion, we should clarify what the words *negative* and *positive* actually mean before we discuss testing. This can be confusing because, although in general speech the word *negative* usually means something bad, with respect to medical tests it means that the problems that were being tested for were not found. The word *positive* means that an abnormality was found. Whether or not a positive test result is good or bad depends on your viewpoint and on the test being run. It can be good that the problem was found, or it can be bad that you have a problem.

The Biopsy

The presence of villous atrophy can be determined by a *biopsy* taken during an *endoscopy*. An endoscopy, basically a scoping or viewing of the intestinal tract, is usually done in a hospital. The patient is heavily medicated and a cable is placed into his or her mouth, down the esophagus, past the stomach, and into the very upper part of the small intestine, known as the *duodenum*. Fiber optics in the cable transmit an image of the gastrointestinal tract to a monitor. This procedure allows the doctor to see inside the esophagus, the stomach, and the duodenum. The endoscope also allows the doctor to place instruments through the cable in order to do things such as takes biopsies.

Villous atrophy cannot be seen with the endoscope; it can be seen only under a microscope. Therefore, a very small cutter is used to remove a tiny piece of tissue, only a few millimeters long, to be examined later. This is called a biopsy. Because villous atrophy can't be seen, the doctor must essentially make an educated guess about where it might be.[10] To increase the likelihood that villous atrophy will be found, at least four to six biopsies should be taken.

After the tissue samples are taken from the patient, they are then sent to the lab. Once at the lab they must be properly oriented on a slide in order to be properly interpreted. And then a *pathologist* well versed in interpreting these types of tissue samples for damage caused by celiac disease must evaluate the slides.

---

10 Note for doctors: Some changes that can be seen in the duodenum during a biopsy are suggestive of celiac disease. These include reduced or absent duodenal folds, scalloping of folds, mosaic pattern to the mucosa, mucosal fissures or cracks, and visible blood vessels. However, there are many other potential causes for these changes, and the duodenum can also appear normal.

Kathy

Kathy was surprised when she was diagnosed with high blood pressure, because she was only 48 and no one in her family had ever had blood pressure problems. At first it was easily controlled by medication, so she didn't worry about it too much.

Over the next several years, she developed several other conditions, including insomnia and a rash that appeared intermittently on her neck, both of which she attributed to stress. She started to feel full all the time but, even though she couldn't eat much at one sitting, she started gaining weight. Her blood pressure increased to the point where the medication that had worked so well in the past was no longer enough to control it. Worst of all, her hip and ankle hurt so badly that when she walked or stood for more than a few minutes, she broke out in a sweat. An MRI showed spinal stenosis, or a narrowing of the spinal column.

While on a trip with her husband, Tom, she awoke one night with chills and nausea. The next day she could barely stay awake. Her sinuses and throat felt swollen. These symptoms came and went over the next few days. On the last day of their vacation, she was so tired and in so much pain that they canceled their sightseeing plans. The day after they got home, they rented her a wheelchair.

Her symptoms continued. About two weeks after their trip, her blood pressure dropped alarmingly and her chest hurt. Scared she might be having a heart attack, she went to the emergency room. The staff there ran tests, determined that her heart was fine, told her that she might have an ulcer, and sent her home.

Her doctor, on the other hand, suspected she might have a virus, but he suggested that she have an endoscopy just in case. A biopsy was also done and to everyone's surprise, it showed that she had celiac disease.

Fortunately for Kathy, her good friend Hayley has celiac disease and helped her establish a gluten-free diet. Within two days, Kathy's nausea was gone. As she got ready to leave work a few days later, she realized with a shock that her hip had hardly bothered her all day. Within a week, she was able to walk and stand more than she had in years, and she returned the wheelchair.

Now, several years later, she no longer takes blood pressure medication. She knows when she's accidentally eaten gluten because she gets a headache, a minor rash, insomnia, or a bit of hip pain, but for the most part she's symptom free. When someone feels sorry for her because she has to follow a gluten-free diet, she says, "Are you kidding? It's given me my life back!"

✦ What Can Go Wrong with the Biopsy

All of this is much easer said than done. A biopsy is a very subjective test because the results are dependent on the experience and interpretation of the doctors and pathologists, and also on luck. There are several places where problems can occur. Let's examine each of them.

First, because the villi are so small, villous atrophy can easily be missed during the biopsy. This is further complicated by the fact that even if it is present, villous atrophy does not necessarily occur consistently throughout the small intestine. It may be patchy, barely there, or in an area that is unreachable by the scope. Therefore, even if the doctor takes six biopsies, there is no guarantee that they are being taken from places where villous atrophy is present.

Second, the biopsy may not be properly interpreted at the lab. Properly orienting the tissue sample on the slide requires some luck, and the pathologist cannot know if it is properly oriented until he or she compares several samples from the same patient. If the sample is not properly oriented, then it may not show villous atrophy even if it is present in the biopsy sample.

Third, the pathologist must be very experienced at determining whether or not the tissue sample actually shows villous atrophy. When the pathologist looks into the microscope, the tissue sample does not necessarily scream "Villous atrophy!" There are varying degrees and severities of damage. Some are very subtle, so that even if everything discussed above has gone well, the presence of villous atrophy may not be spotted.

Finally, if you have not eaten gluten for some time before the biopsy, then the villi will have likely returned to their normal healthy condition. Therefore, even if you have celiac disease, it cannot be diagnosed because the biopsy does not demonstrate villous atrophy. It typically takes several weeks to months of gluten avoidance for this to occur.

✦ Other Potential Causes of a Positive Biopsy

The fact that a biopsy reveals villous atrophy may not mean that you have celiac disease. Villous atrophy can be caused by other conditions. There are documented cases of villous atrophy caused by cow's milk allergy, soy allergy, fish intolerance, chicken intolerance, opportunistic infections, tropical sprue, HIV enteropathy, intestinal lymphoma, ulcerative jejunitis, giardiasis, strongyloidiasis, coccidiosis, hookworm disease, leukemia, intestinal carcinoma, kwashiorkor, methotrexate (a pharmaceutical drug), eosinophilic gastroenteritis (which can be caused by another food allergy or intolerance), and viral gastroenteritis. There are likely other causes which have not yet been discovered.

Although it has traditionally been thought that villous atrophy caused by something other than celiac disease — especially allergies and intolerances to other foods — is exceptionally rare, the reality is that these causes are rarely found because they are rarely looked for. Ironically, this is exactly the same trap that doctors have fallen into when it comes to diagnosing celiac disease. Celiac disease itself was considered rare until we started to look for it. And, although recognition for celiac disease is beginning to grow, it is still rare to evaluate patients properly for dairy or soy allergies or for fish or chicken intolerances (this is discussed in more detail in Chapter 12).

This is not to suggest that if you have been diagnosed with celiac disease following a positive biopsy, you should consider it to be an incorrect diagnosis. Based on everything we know, it is still very likely that it is the correct diagnosis, especially if any of the following tests are positive. However, it is important not to pretend that the biopsy is something other than what it actually is: an imperfect test.

The Tissue Transglutaminase Antibody Test

The second most common test for diagnosing celiac disease is a blood test called the tissue transglutaminase antibody test. Some scientific studies have indicated that it is as effective as the biopsy for determining whether or not a person has villous atrophy. Other studies have suggested that it may produce a negative result in some cases of mild villous atrophy. However, the accuracy of this test (as well as the accuracy of the other blood tests) is always evaluated by how well it performs against the biopsy, since the biopsy has traditionally been considered the gold standard. This is problematic because, as you now know, the biopsy isn't perfect. Attempting to determine the accuracy of one test by comparing it to an imperfect test leaves a lot to be desired. However, this is less problematic than it first appears because, as we will discuss in the next chapter, if someone is diagnosed with a gluten intolerance, specific testing for celiac disease may not be necessary.

As mentioned earlier, tissue transglutaminase is an enzyme that fixes damage in the intestinal tract. When celiac patients ingest gluten, their bodies create an immune response against tissue transglutaminase in the form of *antibodies*, which attack this important enzyme. This is what makes celiac disease an auto-immune disease. Tissue transglutaminase is part of you, and your immune system is attacking it.

The immune system can produce different types of antibodies against tissue transglutaminase, including IgA and IgG antibodies. Because the IgA tissue transglutaminase antibody test is more sensitive for detecting celiac disease and is more readily available than the IgG tissue transglutaminase antibody test, it is more commonly used. The first time any IgA antibody test is run, a total IgA test must also be run, because about 2% of people with celiac disease are IgA deficient. This means that they produce very little IgA and any IgA test result will always be low. For these people, the IgA tissue transglutaminase test can be falsely negative, indicating that they don't have celiac disease even if they in fact do have it. Therefore if the total IgA is below normal, an IgG tissue transglutaminase test can be run instead, to get around the problem of IgA deficiency.

The most common method of measuring the presence of tissue transglutaminase antibodies is to see if they are present in a patient's blood sample by bringing the blood sample in contact with actual transglutaminase enzyme. Any antibodies formed against this enzyme can be measured when they bind to it. The lab may use either the human or guinea pig version of this enzyme. However, tests using the human enzyme are considered more accurate than those using the guinea pig enzyme.

There are reported cases of the tissue transglutaminase test producing positive results due to liver disease, diabetes, severe heart failure, arthritis, and several autoimmune disorders other than celiac disease. However, due to the problems with the biopsy previously discussed, it is difficult to verify that these patients did not truly have celiac disease.

Despite all of this, based on everything that we currently know, in the vast majority of cases if the tissue transglutaminase antibody test is positive, then a diagnosis of celiac disease can be made and a biopsy will not provide any new information on how to treat the patient. If the tissue transglutaminase test is negative, then it is remotely possible that a biopsy will provide a diagnosis of celiac disease, but only if everyone involved in performing and interpreting the samples is very skilled at recognizing mild cases.

If you have not eaten gluten for some time before the test, you will not be producing tissue transglutaminase antibodies even if you are celiac. Therefore there will be no antibodies to be measured and the test will not tell you whether or not you have celiac disease. The exact amount of time for which you must avoid gluten in order for this to happen is unknown, but it is probably a matter of weeks.

Endomysial Antibodies

The endomysial antibody test is an older test. Since it was developed, we have learned that the specific part of the endomysium that is being attacked is the tissue transglutaminase enzyme. Therefore, we can now test specifically for tissue transglutaminase antibodies as we discussed above. Most studies indicate that the tissue transglutaminase test is more reliable for diagnosing celiac disease than the endomysial antibody test. However, the endomysial antibody test is still commonly used and can be useful, with and without other types of testing.

The endomysium is the tissue that lines the intestinal tract. In the endomysial antibody test, the patient's blood is combined with real endomysial tissue. This combination is then observed under the microscope by a lab technician to determine whether or not the blood is triggering a reaction against the endomysium. If it is, then the patient has tested positive for endomysial antibodies.

A positive endomysial antibody test does demonstrate that you have celiac disease. But if the result is negative, it could be a false negative. The tissue transglutaminase IgA antibody test, as well as a total IgA test, should be run to determine whether or not the result was accurate.

As with the tissue transglutaminase antibody test, if you have not eaten gluten for some time, then the endomysial antibody test cannot tell you whether or not you have celiac disease. In addition, the results of the tissue transglutaminase antibody and the endomysial antibody tests depend on the severity of the damage to the small intestine. Therefore, they may be negative when there is only very slight damage to the small intestine, even if it was caused by gluten intolerance. Such minor damage may also be difficult to detect with a biopsy.

There are cases of patients who have a negative endomysial antibody test but a positive tissue transglutaminase test, or a positive endomysial antibody test but a negative tissue transglutaminase test. This may be due to operator error, since the endomysial antibody test is not automated and is highly dependent on the lab technician performing the test. It may also be due to the use of guinea pig tissue transglutaminase (see above). Dr. Peter Green, a noted celiac disease expert, has suggested that because the endo-mysial antibody test is more comprehensive than the tissue trans-glutaminase test, a positive result for endomysial antibodies always indicates a gluten intolerance, even if the tissue transglutaminase test or a biopsy is negative. This seems to be a logical conclusion.

Reticulin Antibodies

Reticulin antibody testing is truly outdated, yet it is still often run. Reticular cells are found in connective tissues, especially those of the lymphatic system, and are common along the digestive tract. Reticulin antibodies are formed to attack reticular cells. These antibodies are not specific to celiac disease or gluten intolerance. Reticulin antibody testing misses the diagnosis of celiac disease too frequently to be considered worth running now that we have much better tests.

Gliadin Antibodies

Gliadin antibodies cannot be used to determine whether or not you have celiac disease. However, they are very useful for determining if you have another form of gluten intolerance. They will be discussed in the next chapter on non-celiac forms of gluten intolerance.

Stool Testing for Antibodies

A few labs offer stool testing for one or more of the antibodies mentioned above. Stool testing evaluates the presence of secretory IgA antibodies (sIgA), or IgA antibodies secreted into the digestive tract, which are somewhat different than the IgA antibodies found in the blood. There are very few studies on the usefulness of stool testing for celiac antibodies and those that exist have come to very different conclusions about its accuracy. Unfortunately, each of the existing studies was poorly designed and it is difficult to glean much practical information from them. There are no studies that compare the presence of sIgA antibodies with blood IgA antibodies.

Although there are some advocates of stool testing for antibodies to diagnose celiac disease and gluten intolerance, there is little scientific evidence at this time to support using this type of testing. However, this does not prove that it is invalid, and it should be noted that many people feel that they have been significantly helped by stool testing. More research into this area is warranted.

Salivary Testing for Antibodies

Salivary testing for one or more of the antibodies mentioned in this chapter has the same problem as stool testing. The very few studies on the subject have come to different conclusions, and it is therefore difficult to evaluate this type of testing. However, the studies seem to indicate that if the test shows that the antibody is present in the saliva, then it is an accurate result. But if the antibody is not found in the saliva, it may still be found in the bloodstream, making it likely that saliva testing often produces false negative results.

Genetic Testing

Much has been written about genetic testing for celiac disease and it is easy to get excited about anything related to genetics. However, genetic testing for celiac disease isn't nearly the pot of gold at the end of the rainbow that many people hoped it would be. In fact, genetic testing has only limited value when it comes to predicting whether or not someone has celiac disease or will get celiac disease. Let's take a closer look at this issue.

Two genes have been primarily associated with celiac disease: HLA-DQ2 and HLA-DQ8. Most people with celiac disease have these genes, but not all of them do. However, approximately 30% of the population have these genes. Since we know that it is *not* true that 30% of the population have celiac disease, then we know that having these genes cannot predict whether or not you have or will get celiac disease.

Therefore, genetic testing does not tell you anything about your condition. If you already know that you have celiac disease, then you won't learn anything from genetic testing. If you do not know for sure whether you have it, genetic testing will not give you the answer. If you don't have it, you cannot use genetic testing to predict whether or not you will get it. And remember, *nearly* all people with celiac disease have these genes, but some do not. In addition, because no research has been done on genetic testing for other forms of gluten intolerance, millions of people who have a non-celiac form of gluten intolerance may not have these genes.

Using genetic testing for celiac disease is almost like saying that everyone with celiac disease has either an X or a Y chromosome. And what does that tell you? Not much — at least not at this time.

Genes are far more complicated than they are portrayed in the media. An excellent cover article in *Discover*, "DNA Is Not Destiny," pointed out that in most cases merely having a particular gene does not determine what will happen to you. Genes require instructions that tell them what to do, that turn them either on or off. Instructions come from the environment in the form of vitamins, foods, toxins, stress, and literally everything we do and are exposed to. All of these things affect our genetic expression. This fascinating lesson tells us that we are not necessarily at the mercy of our genes. In fact, our genes are also at the mercy of our actions and environment. It's definitely food for thought.

Confocal Laser Endomicroscopy

A new development in the endoscopy world is called confocal laser endomicroscopy. The makers of this equipment claim that it allows a doctor to make a diagnosis of celiac disease *during* an endoscopy by taking very detailed microscopic pictures of the cells of the intestinal tract, thus avoiding the need for a biopsy. The doctor can evaluate as many tissue samples as needed while performing the procedure, without actually cutting any tissue. Therefore the diagnosis of villous atrophy and, thus, of celiac disease can be made on the spot. This technology may one day eliminate the biopsy, but it won't eliminate the endoscopy procedure. It is not yet widely available.

Camera in a Capsule

It is now possible to swallow a camera in a capsule. The camera takes images of your intestinal tract as it passes through. While this test can see large abnormalities of the intestinal tract, such as ulcers and polyps, it does not diagnose celiac disease, gluten intolerance, or other food sensitivities.

MRI, CT Scan, X-Ray, and Ultrasound

The MRI, CT scan, X-ray, and ultrasound are diagnostic tools commonly used to assess patients who have digestive or abdominal problems. However, they are not capable of determining whether or not someone has celiac disease or a gluten intolerance.

Colonoscopy

The colonoscopy is an examination of the colon using a fiber-optic scope. It is another useful diagnostic tool with many worthwhile functions. However, it does not have any value in diagnosing celiac disease or gluten intolerance.

Fecal Fat

People with celiac disease often have a problem absorbing the fat in their diet. This is called *steatorrhea*. Not being able to absorb fat may sound like a good thing, but ultimately it is very unhealthy. Doctors will sometimes run a test to measure the amount of fat found in a stool sample. While this can be informative, all it says is that there is fat in your stool. This test does not determine the cause of the fat in the stool, and there are many potential causes.

Intestinal Permeability

Tests that measure intestinal permeability (leaky gut), such as the xylose test and the lactulose test, are used to determine if an unusually high level of a substance — more than would normally be expected — is being absorbed by the digestive tract. These tests are not specific to any one condition, but simply determine whether there is inflammation and damage in the digestive tract that would lead to an increase in the number and size of the molecules that are being absorbed across the intestinal wall. If the results are positive, the question still remains: What is causing the increase in intestinal permeability? Celiac disease can be a cause, as can gluten intolerance, reactions to other foods, and many other conditions. Therefore tests that measure intestinal permeability have very limited value, because they don't offer much information on how to treat the cause of the problem.

The Biopsy as the Gold Standard?

The biopsy is considered the gold standard test for celiac disease. It has been the preferred method of diagnosing celiac disease for several decades. Amazingly enough, the quality of all other tests for celiac disease are measured against the biopsy. If a test is considered good, it is because it agrees with the biopsy. If a test is considered bad, it is because it does not agree with the biopsy. Yet it is evident that the biopsy is fraught with potential for human error.

By this point you should be asking yourself, "How can this be?" If a doctor has a choice between a test that requires a simple blood draw or one that requires sedation for a hospital procedure, doesn't it make sense to go for the easiest and least traumatic method? Well, doctors are human, and it's not always easy to change human behavior. They are accustomed to using the biopsy rather than a blood test. The biopsy is a complicated procedure and brings in a lot more money than a blood test. It's also visual and, all too often in medicine, seeing is believing. When you go to the doctor with a digestive problem, it is likely that most of the tests he or she orders will be visual: endoscopy, colonoscopy, CT scan, X-ray, MRI, and ultrasound.

Unfortunately, the intestinal biopsy is often done when there is no practical reason to do one. This is especially true *after* the diagnosis of celiac disease. It is common to recommend that a follow-up biopsy be done several months or a year after the original diagnosis of celiac disease, supposedly to determine whether or not the patient is healing. But the results of the follow-up biopsy have no impact on the outcome of the patient. They don't change the treatment plan, they don't improve healing, and they don't predict or prevent any future problems. In fact, one could easily argue that this procedure interferes with the healing process. Whether or not the patient's villi are returning to normal can be interesting, and there are times when having that information may be valuable, but usually this is for scientific purposes. A patient's healing progress can usually be monitored based on his or her symptoms. If the patient is not healing properly, then many other issues should be considered; these will be discussed later in this book. However, performing another endoscopy within a year or two is unlikely to shed further light on the situation with regard to celiac disease.

With all of the emphasis placed on the biopsy, it is somewhat ironic that most of the studies to determine how common celiac disease is in the general population were based on blood tests. Even more telling, in some studies a biopsy was performed after the blood test to demonstrate that the blood test was correct. In most cases there is little to be gained by performing a biopsy once a blood test has already made a determination of celiac disease.

What Is the Treatment for Celiac Disease?

The treatment for celiac disease is to stop eating gluten. This is easier said than done, but many thousands of people find that they are capable of completely removing gluten from their diet. Of course, it does take conscious effort. Gluten is found in almost all bread products, pastas, soy sauce, and many, many processed foods. However, many companies are now producing an ever-increasing number of gluten-free alternatives. This topic will be explored in more detail in the chapter on treating gluten intolerance.

What Is the Long-Term Outcome for People with Celiac Disease?

Fortunately, removing gluten from the diet usually reverses the intestinal damage that has already occurred. Most people notice significant improvement within weeks, if not days, and may continue to heal for one to two years. However, healing time can vary and may take months. It also tends to vary with age. As with most conditions, the older the patient, the slower the recovery.

Dermatitis Herpetiformis: Celiac Disease of the Skin?

A skin condition called dermatitis herpetiformis, or DH, is often considered to be another form of celiac disease because it is triggered by the ingestion of gluten. Those with DH experience extreme itching and usually a blistering rash. These often occur on the elbows and knees, but can be anywhere on the body. Sufferers may scratch until their skin breaks or bleeds.

DH is traditionally diagnosed by evaluating a biopsy of the skin for IgA deposits under the top layer of skin. As with the intestinal biopsy, it is a subjective test and it can be very difficult to get the correct biopsy of the correct tissue. In fact, IgA deposits are not measurable in the blisters, but only in the few millimeters next to a blister. We know that, due to the limitations of the biopsy, not everyone with DH will have a positive skin biopsy.

If you have DH, it does not necessarily mean that you have villous atrophy in your intestine. Only around 80% of people with DH test positive for celiac disease, meaning that about 20% do not have villous atrophy. When the results of the skin biopsy were originally discovered to correlate fairly closely with those of the biopsy of the small intestine, DH was classified as a form of celiac disease. However, it is obvious that the two are not the same and do not occur simultaneously or at the same rate.

DH is an excellent example of a symptom other than villous atrophy that can result from gluten intolerance. It has been so narrowly defined that by definition it can be triggered only by a gluten intolerance. However, other skin problems (as mentioned in the previous chapter), including some causing itchiness, may also be triggered by gluten, but because they have triggers other than a gluten intolerance, they cannot be thought of as being so closely linked to celiac disease. DH, like villous atrophy, is a symptom, not a disease. This is why DH properly fits in the list of symptoms associated with gluten intolerance in Chapter 3.

Summary

Celiac disease is defined by a type of damage that can occur in the small intestine of someone with a gluten intolerance. This damage is called villous atrophy. Therefore celiac disease is a symptom, synonymous with villous atrophy. The tissue transglutaminase antibody test, a blood test, is generally very good for diagnosing celiac disease, as is the intestinal biopsy. However, the intestinal biopsy is an overused diagnostic tool that often does not add new information to what can be learned from a simple blood test.

Questions remain about the validity of each of these tests, and there is a distinct possibility that causes other than gluten intolerance can lead to a positive test result. A great deal more research needs to done on other potential causes of villous atrophy and their effects on both the biopsy and the blood tests. Interestingly, the European standard for diagnosing celiac disease requires both a positive biopsy *and* improvement in the patient's condition after eliminating gluten from his or her diet. This standard was developed with the clear understanding that villous atrophy by itself is not complete proof of gluten intolerance. This is true whether villous atrophy is diagnosed with a biopsy or a blood test. (This standard also indicates that if you have been diagnosed with celiac disease and are avoiding gluten but not getting better, then you should seek out more information about why you are not well. This is discussed in Chapter 12.)

Still, in spite of the potential confusion and problems associated with the various tests for diagnosing celiac disease, the most highly recognized tests are generally very good and should continue to be used and respected. Fortunately, most of the pitfalls associated with them can be avoided if we simply step back and take a look at the bigger picture — gluten intolerance, which is not necessarily the same as celiac disease. This will be discussed in the next chapter.

part III

Non-Celiac Gluten Intolerance and Wheat Allergies

The Untold Story: Understanding and Testing for Non-Celiac Forms of Gluten Intolerance

*Discovery is to see what everyone else has seen
and to think what no one else has thought.*
— 1937 Nobel Prize winner Albert Szent-Györgyi (1893–1986)

*Do you remember how electrical currents
and "unseen waves" were laughed at?
The knowledge about man is still in its infancy.*
— Albert Einstein (1879–1955)

In this chapter we look at the many forms of gluten intolerance that do not fit the definition of celiac disease. This is possibly the most important chapter in this book. While much has been written about celiac disease, little has been written about non-celiac forms of gluten intolerance, despite the fact that there are far more people who find that they react to gluten than can be accounted for by celiac disease. Although celiac disease gets most of the media and medical attention, millions of people who are gluten intolerant don't qualify for a diagnosis of celiac disease.

This whole concept of *non-celiac gluten intolerance* may be new to you. You might be asking, "Aren't celiac disease and gluten intolerance the same thing?" The short answer is "no." Many people who cannot tolerate gluten have been thoroughly tested for celiac disease and it is clear that they do not have it.

Some of you might be saying, "How can this possibly be?" Others are probably saying, "It's about time someone acknowledged this." You may know from personal experience that you have a gluten intolerance, but your doctor has told you that you do not have celiac disease. And your doctor was probably correct. Assuming that the proper testing was done and that it was done accurately, as discussed in the previous chapter, it is highly unlikely that you have celiac disease.

It is important to point out right away that these other forms of gluten intolerance are no less significant or less harmful than celiac disease. The idea that non-celiac gluten intolerance is less important than celiac disease is a common but mistaken assumption that we will discuss further in this chapter.

The Difference Between Celiac Disease and Other Forms of Gluten Intolerance

So what is the difference between celiac disease and non-celiac forms of gluten intolerance? In the previous chapter we established that celiac disease is defined by villous atrophy, a very specific type of damage to the small intestine. If you do not have villous atrophy, then you do not have celiac disease. Celiac disease and villous atrophy are essentially one and the same. This is an extremely important point. Celiac disease is not only defined by villous atrophy, it *is* villous atrophy.

However, many potential problems can result from a gluten intolerance. Villous atrophy is only one of these; therefore, *celiac disease is only one form of gluten intolerance among many*. It does not encompass or define gluten intolerance.

The other important point to understand is that once villous atrophy has been diagnosed, the damage has already been done.

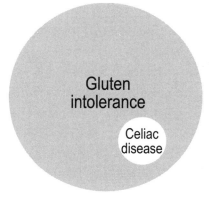

Figure 3. The Relationship Between
Gluten Intolerance and Celiac Disease

Removing gluten from the diet can have impressive results in improving your health, but the illness may have led to other damage that is irreversible. Even villous atrophy, which is usually thought of as reversible, is in many cases not so, especially in older patients.

It is not necessary to wait for villous atrophy to develop to determine if gluten is damaging your health. It and many other problems can be prevented by testing for the broader problem of gluten intolerance.

Is Celiac Disease Worse than Other Forms of Gluten Intolerance?

People often mistakenly assume that celiac disease is the worst form of gluten intolerance and that if you don't have celiac disease, then you don't really have to worry about your gluten intolerance as much as you would if you had been diagnosed with celiac disease. This idea is unfortunately perpetuated by the medical community, but it is also inherent in the use of the word *disease*. Celiac is not a disease in the popular sense of the word. It is not a bacteria or a virus, nor is it contagious. It is simply a reaction to a food. We don't even use this type of strong label for life-threatening food allergies, which are far more dangerous in the short term than celiac disease.

Certainly, celiac disease can become so severe that it puts people's lives in danger. It can inhibit the absorption of nutrients so much that sufferers fail to absorb anything they eat. They may lose weight and become dehydrated to the point that they can barely sustain themselves and end up in the hospital. Such dramatic cases do occur, but they do not necessarily describe what happens to the average person with celiac disease. In fact, they do not even describe an inevitable end stage of celiac disease, much less of gluten intolerance.

Many people who have celiac disease do not suffer from noticeable symptoms for many years. They may live almost their entire lives without any real health problems or, more likely, they may have relatively minor health issues related to an unrecognized gluten intolerance. But then they are diagnosed with, for example, osteoporosis, and a discerning physician discovers that they have celiac disease. Or they develop colon cancer and it is discovered that they have celiac disease. These people didn't just suddenly develop celiac disease. They had a gluten intolerance all their lives. Yet kids can have celiac disease too, and many are so sick that they exhibit what is called "failure to thrive." They are not absorbing the nutrition from their food and, therefore, they do not gain weight, do not grow, and lack energy. Most people fall somewhere in the middle, suffering from some type of problem but not getting properly diagnosed.

It is clear that celiac disease can range from mild to severe and that it can be severe at any age. The flip side of this is that many people with a non-celiac gluten intolerance have tremendous health problems. Again we refer back to the list of potential symptoms and conditions in Chapter 3. These are associated with *gluten intolerance*, not just celiac disease.

You may have terrible diarrhea triggered by gluten, yet not have celiac disease. Your child may experience poor growth or poor attention caused by a gluten intolerance, yet not have celiac disease. You may be chronically anemic (iron deficient) due to a gluten intolerance, but not have celiac disease. The list goes on and on. The bottom line is that you may suffer from one of the many problems that can result from a gluten intolerance, but not have villous atrophy.

Ironically, every year thousands of people go to hospital emergency rooms because they are suffering from severe abdominal pain or other digestive problems. For a tremendous number of these people, it turns out that they do *not* have appendicitis, gallbladder problems, ulcers, celiac disease, or any other known problem. They are given no good explanation for their suffering and are simply sent home with pain medication. Many of these people are suffering from a gluten intolerance.

The symptoms that one person with a non-celiac gluten intolerance experiences may be much worse than those of another person with celiac disease. Or it may be the other way around. Gluten intolerance, whether or not it is celiac disease, can range from mild to severe.

Is Celiac Disease the End Stage of Gluten Intolerance?

It is often assumed that celiac disease is the final result of gluten intolerance. This is probably related to the assumption that celiac disease is the worst form of gluten intolerance and the most life-threatening form. Neither of these assumptions is based on what we actually know about celiac disease.

Will you eventually get celiac disease (villous atrophy) if you are gluten intolerant and you continue to eat gluten? We don't know the answer to this question. Because so much of the research is focused on celiac disease, very little is known about the development of other forms of gluten intolerance. But is it really all that important? Either way, damage is being done to the body and the consequences can be significant. People who are gluten intolerant should be strongly advised to avoid gluten. Whether or not they could eventually develop celiac disease is not the main issue. The consequences can be severe in either case.

What Are the Symptoms of Non-Celiac Gluten Intolerance?

If you refer back to the list of conditions associated with gluten intolerance in Chapter 3, you'll notice that villous atrophy is just one of many types of damage that can be caused by gluten intolerance. Most of the other conditions apply to both celiac and non-celiac gluten intolerance. But villous atrophy (celiac disease) does not have to be present to experience most of these other problems. As listed in Chapter 3, the most common symptoms of gluten intolerance are these:

- Diarrhea
- Constipation
- Heartburn
- Abdominal pain
- Headaches (including migraines)
- Fatigue
- Muscle aches
- Joint pain
- Hypoglycemia
- Eczema
- Acne
- Mental fogginess
- Anemia (iron or B12 deficiency)
- Frequent illness
- Itchy skin
- Low bone density

While many people may think of gluten intolerance primarily as
a digestive problem, you can see that it has the potential to affect
almost every part of the body.

How Many People Have Non-Celiac Gluten Intolerance?

Many people, probably many millions of people, have a non-
celiac form of gluten intolerance and experience one or more
of these problems. Because the conditions associated with non-
celiac gluten intolerance have more than one potential cause, and
because so little research has been done on non-celiac forms of
gluten intolerance, it is difficult to say how often these symptoms
are caused by a gluten intolerance. It is possible that gluten intolerance is the cause far more often than most people currently
suspect.[11] Recent studies estimate that non-celiac forms of gluten
intolerance are approximately 30 times more common than celiac
disease and may affect up to 15% of the world's population.

What Goes Wrong for These People When They See the Doctor?

Many doctors still do not have a very good appreciation for celiac
disease and often fail to test for it, even when the patient has
the traditional symptoms of diarrhea and bloating. This lack of
awareness is magnified hundreds of times when we're discussing
the broader topic of non-celiac gluten intolerance. Extremely few
physicians understand that non-celiac forms of gluten intolerance
exist. If the patient has a negative test for celiac disease, then most
physicians would consider that this result rules out all gluten intolerance and not pursue the issue any further.

---

11 If we expand this discussion to include foods other than gluten, the
author believes that in a tremendous number of cases we will find that
these health problems are caused by reactions to food.

Other tests likely to be run include a colonoscopy, endoscopy, parasite testing, standard blood tests, and possibly even an X-ray, ultrasound, MRI, or CT scan. But none of these tests are capable of diagnosing a non-celiac gluten intolerance. After a lot of time and what might seem like a very thorough set of tests and exams, the patient is still left without an answer. He or she may be given medications in an attempt to alter the symptoms, but no hope for understanding what's behind the symptoms or how to truly cure the problem. Some doctors will even blame stress or anxiety, which, unfortunately, can lead patients to believe that the problem is all in their head. But nothing could be further from the truth.

If doctors only knew how to test for non-celiac intolerance, then they could save many people a tremendous amount of suffering. Although most doctors aren't familiar with testing for non-celiac gluten intolerance, the irony is that the test is a fairly simple one that many of them are already running without even knowing that it can diagnose this problem. In fact, as many people have already learned, you can sometimes even determine for yourself if you have a gluten intolerance. Both of these topics will be discussed in the next section.

Grace

If you met Grace now, she'd seem like a typical 15-year-old. She loves to play soccer and hang out with her friends. But just a few short years ago, Grace's life was very different. She suffered from diarrhea, frequent headaches, and eczema, which were distressing and caused her to miss many days of school. As she got older, she started to experience severe fatigue and at the age of 11 was diagnosed with vitamin B12 deficiency anemia.

Because Grace's mother and two older siblings have all been diagnosed with celiac disease, Grace was tested every year when she was younger. Despite her typical celiac symptoms, the tests continued to come back negative until she was 12 years old, when she finally tested positive.

While they were relieved to find the source of Grace's health problems — and are thrilled that she leads a happier and more active life now that she's on a gluten-free diet — her parents are worried about how the years of malabsorption and inflammation she suffered as a child might affect her in the future. They wish that they had been informed about non-celiac gluten intolerance and that she had been tested for it, not just celiac disease, at a younger age. By avoiding gluten earlier, she would have had a happier and healthier childhood and would have avoided developing celiac disease at all.

Finding Out If You Have a Non-Celiac Gluten Intolerance

There are several ways to determine if you are gluten intolerant. Some are easier than others, depending on your point of view, but they are not equally reliable. In this section we will discuss the different methods and their advantages and disadvantages.

Elimination Diets

Many people figure out that they are gluten intolerant by themselves. Suspecting that gluten is causing their problems, they simply avoid it and then feel much better. There is nothing wrong with this approach, but it is not necessarily well received by doctors. It is shocking how often doctors ignore this feedback from their patients. Worse yet, some healthcare providers give their patients the impression that by not eating wheat, they are depriving themselves of something so nutritious that they can't possibly be healthy. This is, of course, absurd. Millions of people on this planet don't eat wheat and are very healthy, as we discussed in Chapter 1. Other doctors simply don't like it when people diagnose themselves with a food reaction. Maybe they feel threatened by this. Whatever the reason, remember that your doctor provides a valuable service, but you are the owner of your body. Don't let a healthcare professional tell you that you can't possibly know what is good for you.

While elimination diets can be useful, they are also tricky. Eliminating gluten from your diet can be very difficult and time consuming. First, you need to have a complete understanding of gluten and all the various processed foods that can contain it (see Chapter 9). Second, assuming that you are able to avoid *all* gluten *all* the time, it may still take several weeks or months for your body to heal and for you to notice improvement.

Finally, gluten may not be the cause of your problem, or it may be only part of the cause, in which case you may fail to notice any improvement in your health. Or any improvement you do notice might not be due to your avoidance of wheat and gluten. When you eliminate these foods, you may also inadvertently avoid other foods that you eat with them, thereby confusing the issue. For example, bread often contains dairy products and other ingredients as well as wheat, and it almost always contains baker's yeast. Or, as another example, maybe you tend to eat cheese (dairy) or mayo (egg) with your bread, and when you stop eating bread you do not eat them either.

You should also be aware that, as with testing for celiac disease, eliminating gluten from your diet will make it difficult to test for gluten intolerance. After a few weeks of avoiding gluten, your

test results will be normal even if they would have been positive
if you were still eating gluten. Of course, if you are in doubt about
the impact that gluten is having on your health, you can reintroduce it for a month or more and then start testing.

Blood Tests for Diagnosing Non-Celiac Gluten Intolerance

Fortunately, you generally don't have to rely on experimenting with
your diet to find out if you have a non-celiac gluten intolerance. At
the Innate Health Group's IBS Treatment Center, tests for gluten
intolerance and other food allergies and intolerances are routinely
run before starting people on a treatment plan and making any
changes in their diet. However, when it comes specifically to
testing for a gluten intolerance, any physician can do that if he or
she so desires, and many often do so without even realizing it.

There are very specific scientific ways to test for non-celiac
gluten intolerance. Recall from Chapter 4 that when the immune
system attacks a food in a person with a food intolerance, it cre-
ates antibodies. Blood tests can measure these antibodies. When
done properly, this type of testing is extremely valuable and can
be used to measure immune reactions to any food. The immune
system does not form an antibody reaction against a food unless
there is a problem with that food. In the case of non-celiac gluten
intolerance, we are looking for antibodies that attack gluten or a
particular grain, such as wheat, barley, or rye.

This is different from testing for antibodies that are specific to
just one type of damage, such as villous atrophy, which is how we
test for celiac disease. In order to see the bigger picture, we need to
broaden our approach and look for an antibody that is evidence
of the entire range of gluten intolerance. Fortunately, there is such
an antibody. It is called the *gliadin antibody.*

✦ Food Antibodies as Markers for Health

It is important to address the idea that antibodies targeting food and food components are relevant to health. A person's immune system does not generate antibodies against foods without potential consequences for that person. Three facts support this concept. First, we know that researchers often use the gliadin antibody as a screening tool when investigating celiac disease. It is valuable because it has meaning — it helps narrow down the field of potential candidates for celiac disease. If everyone had elevated antibodies to gliadin then the test would be of no use. Second, studies on other health conditions continue to demonstrate the relevance of these types of antibody reactions (some of these studies are listed in the bibliography of this book).

Third, and most importantly, doctors who test patients for antibody reactions to food and then properly educate their patients on how to avoid foods for which they have elevated antibody levels can see for themselves the dramatic improvement in their patients. But in order for this to happen, the proper tests must be run, the lab work must be of high quality, the physician has to keep in mind all of the possible symptoms that can be triggered by the food (as does the patient), and the food must be eliminated for a long enough period of time for healing to take place. These are the exact same issues at play when diagnosing celiac disease. Of course, if you don't run the tests, or you don't apply the test results, then you won't see their significance. And remember, just because you don't have any bothersome symptoms doesn't mean you aren't reacting to the food. The same issue is also often the case for people with celiac disease.

✦ Testing for Gliadin Antibodies

We mentioned in Chapter 2 that gliadin is a type of gluten. When the immune system attacks gluten, it produces gliadin antibodies. If you have gliadin antibodies, then it is apparent that your immune system has interpreted that gluten is not food; it is a foreign invader that must be eliminated from the body. It attacks any gluten you eat.

We can test for gliadin antibodies with a blood test called the gliadin antibody test. Ironically, this test is often run before or along with the tests for celiac disease. Unfortunately, most doctors don't pay much attention to its result or tend to overlook its value. Even if the gliadin antibody test is positive, they feel that this result is not of much importance unless celiac testing is also positive. If celiac testing is negative, then the gliadin test result is generally considered a false positive or an anomaly, and it is ignored.

Remember, gliadin antibodies are not specific for villous atrophy. Therefore this test cannot be used to test for celiac disease. But it has tremendous value if you are looking for a gluten intolerance because gliadin antibodies are a measure of the immune system's response to gliadin, a type of gluten, which is in wheat and other grains. If the immune system is forming antibodies against gliadin, then it is reacting against these foods and the gliadin antibody test can measure this reaction.

There are primarily three different types of gliadin antibodies of interest: the IgA, IgG, and IgE gliadin antibodies. *Ig* stands for *immunoglobulin*, which is another word for antibody. The three antibodies are different ways in which the immune system can react to something, in this case gluten (gliadin). IgA and IgG gliadin antibodies are the ones most typically tested for by doctors and the ones in which we are most interested when it comes to gluten intolerance. IgE gliadin antibodies will be discussed in the next chapter on conventional IgE gluten and wheat allergies.

If either your IgA or IgG gliadin antibody test is positive, then you have a strong immune reaction to gluten and thus a gluten intolerance. The IgA gliadin antibody test tends to be the more sensitive, but for reasons yet unknown (immunology is still a very young science) the immune system may respond with IgA, IgG, or both antibodies. Any of these reactions is a clear indication that your body is attacking gluten.

✦ Testing for Antibodies Against Gluten-Containing Grains

Far less common, but equally informative, are tests for antibodies formed against any of the gluten-containing grains, such as wheat, barley, rye, and spelt. These tests look for an immune reaction against the food as a whole, rather than against a specific protein, such as gluten (gliadin). These also come in the form of IgA, IgG, and IgE antibody tests. Only a few specialized laboratories run these types of tests, and even fewer do a good job of running them accurately and providing reproducible results.

If you have a positive test result for a gliadin antibody, then you will usually also have a positive test result for antibodies against wheat, barley, rye, spelt, and other gluten-containing grains. However, a positive gliadin antibody test does not guarantee a positive test result for antibodies against *all* of these grains. Wheat and spelt are very closely related and have a very high amount of gluten; therefore, their tests are almost always positive when the gliadin antibody test is positive. However, the further a grain is from wheat on the family tree (see Chapter 2), the smaller the amount of gluten it contains.

Therefore, you may have a negative test result for barley or rye, even though you have a gluten intolerance. This does not mean that you can eat those foods. The test measures the antibody reaction against the whole grain, not the just the gluten (gliadin) component of it. If you do eat barley or rye, you will digest them into their individual proteins and release the gluten contained in them, which will then be attacked by your gliadin (gluten) antibodies.

It is also possible to react to wheat or the other grains without reacting to gluten. You could have a reaction against one of
the many other components in these grains. In this case, you may
have a very strong reaction to the grain in spite of a low reaction
to gliadin. This will be discussed further in the next chapter.

✦ Total IgA

As discussed in Chapter 4, the first time any IgA antibody test is
run, a total IgA test must also be run. About 1% of the population is
IgA deficient (versus 2% of celiacs), meaning that they produce very
little IgA. For these people, any IgA test result will be low, and therefore the IgA gliadin antibody test might be falsely negative, indicating that they don't have a gluten intolerance even if they do.

If your total IgA is below normal, then an IgG gliadin antibody
test can be used to get around the problem of the IgA deficiency.

Biopsy of the Small Intestine

As we discussed in Chapter 4, the biopsy is useful in finding villous
atrophy and thereby diagnosing celiac disease. However, because
other forms of gluten intolerance do not cause villous atrophy, a
negative biopsy result does not rule them out.

Stool Testing for Antibodies

Food antibodies, including gliadin antibodies, may be found in a
person's feces. These are secretory IgA antibodies, also known as
sIgA. These antibodies are somewhat different from the IgA antibodies found in the blood and they are still poorly understood.

There are very few studies on the usefulness of stool testing
for food antibodies and those that exist have come to very different
conclusions about its accuracy. There are no studies that compare
the presence of sIgA antibodies with blood IgA antibodies.

Although there are some advocates for using stool testing for diagnosing gluten intolerance, there is little scientific evidence at this time to support its use. However, that does not prove that it is invalid, and it should be noted that many people feel that they have been significantly helped by stool testing for sIgA antibodies to food. More research into this area is warranted.

Salivary Testing for Antibodies

As with stool testing, little is known about salivary testing for gliadin antibodies. The very few studies on the subject have come to different conclusions, and it is therefore difficult to evaluate this type of testing. However, the studies seem to indicate that if the test shows that the antibody is present in the saliva, then it is an accurate result. But they also suggest that if the antibody is not found in the saliva, it may still be found in the bloodstream, making it appear that saliva testing produces false negative results. Far better tests exist, making salivary testing of little value at this time.

Skin Testing

Skin testing is the type of testing done by most allergy specialists. We know that skin testing for food allergies has no value when it comes to testing for celiac disease, and little if any value in testing for other forms of gluten intolerance. Skin testing measures only IgE antibody-type reactions, and neither celiac disease nor most gluten intolerances cause the production of a measurable amount of IgE antibodies. Neither do other food intolerances, which should make it apparent that skin testing has little value for diagnosing them.

Interestingly, even though skin testing is supposed to measure IgE antibodies, its results do not always correlate very well with those of blood tests that directly measure IgE antibodies. In fact, skin testing misses a large percentage of IgE food reactions. Why is this? Skin testing measures *wheals*, or inflammation of the skin. This inflammation, however, is only one potential symptom of an immune reaction to food. Food allergies, even if we limit our discussion to only IgE-caused reactions, can cause a wide variety of symptoms, not all of which can be measured with skin testing.

This is essentially the same problem that we have been discussing with regard to testing for villous atrophy. Villous atrophy is only one potential reaction to gluten. But a gluten intolerance can trigger a wide range of symptoms, and testing for villous atrophy alone cannot rule out the presence of a gluten intolerance. Even more unfortunately, most allergy specialists fail to test for either celiac disease or gluten intolerance, even though it is well warranted in many of their patients. This is an important fact to know, since it is easy to assume that an allergy specialist would be well versed on these topics.

Summary

Gluten intolerance is a much broader issue than just celiac disease (villous atrophy). You do not need to test positive for celiac disease to have a gluten intolerance. If your biopsy or blood tests are negative for celiac disease, this does not rule out the possibility that you have another form of gluten intolerance. Millions of people suffer from gluten intolerance but do not have celiac disease.

Determining whether or not you have a gluten intolerance can sometimes be done without medical testing, by eliminating gluten from your diet and noticing that you feel much better. Although this can be challenging, many people have discovered their gluten intolerance by doing just this. But if that doesn't work for you, or if you didn't notice any difference when you avoided gluten, or if you are not sure that gluten is really a problem and would like to see a lab result first before you deprive yourself of gluten-containing foods, then there are several lab tests that can be used to assist you.

Ironically, many physicians are already using the primary test for gluten intolerance, the gliadin antibody test. However, most use it only as a stepping-stone to further testing for celiac disease. But if your gliadin antibody test is positive, then you've got your answer. You are gluten intolerant. You can also use blood tests to determine whether or not you have IgG antibodies for wheat, rye, barley, spelt, and other gluten grains, as well as many other foods. The tests will tell you if you are reactive to those foods.

CHAPTER 6

Conventional Wheat Allergies and Non-Gluten Wheat Reactions

Health is the greatest gift, contentment the greatest wealth, faithfulness the best relationship.

—Buddha (Siddhartha Gautama [c. 563–c. 483 B.C.], the founder of Buddhism)

This book is primarily about what can best be described as chronic food intolerances, reactions to wheat and gluten that, although they might be more accurately called *gluten allergies*, do not fit the conventional use of the word *allergy*. However, there are reactions to wheat and to gluten that *do* fit the traditional definition of an allergy. In addition, there are reactions to wheat that do not involve gluten. We will discuss both of these types of reactions in this chapter.

Conventional Wheat and Gluten Allergies

Most people, when they think of an allergy, usually think of an immediate reaction that causes some type of noticeable swelling. This type of reaction is typically triggered by IgE antibodies that ultimately lead to the release of histamine. This is what is meant by a conventional allergy. It is the type of allergy for which your typical allergy doctor is looking.

These kinds of allergies can lead to symptoms such as hives, swollen lips, or even a swollen tongue. They may also cause contact dermatitis, itchiness, and respiratory effects such as asthma. Allergic reactions are known to occur not only in response to the ingestion of wheat and gluten, but also to inhaled wheat flour or gluten and to the application of skin and hair products that contain wheat or gluten, such as shampoos, lotions, and even cosmetics.

Another possible allergic reaction to wheat or gluten is *anaphylaxis*, a condition usually associated with other foods, such as peanuts or shellfish. It is an immediate and body-wide IgE reaction caused by the release of histamines. Anaphylaxis generally involves an exaggerated allergic response that includes both the circulatory and respiratory systems and can potentially be very severe or even life threatening. Symptoms may include swelling, itchiness, low blood pressure, bronchospasm, airway obstruction, edema, shock, loss of consciousness, and ultimately death if medical care is not received in a timely fashion.

People who have any of these types of conventional allergic reactions to the gluten in wheat should avoid all forms of gluten, including barley, rye, spelt, and other gluten-containing grains, just as they would if they had a gluten intolerance.

Skin prick testing is the traditional way to test for these types of food allergies. It is much more successful at diagnosing these conventional allergies than it is at finding the food intolerances that are the main focus of this book. Blood tests may also be used to test for conventional allergies because these allergies produce IgE antibodies that are measurable in the blood. The following results would be found in someone who has a conventional IgE gluten allergy but does not have a gluten intolerance or celiac disease:

IgA and IgG gliadin antibody — negative

IgA and IgG tissue transglutaminase antibody (celiac test)
— negative

IgE wheat antibody — positive

IgE gluten antibody — positive (unless the wheat allergy
does not involve gluten; see below.)

However, as with the other tests previously discussed, if you
do not eat gluten then it is unlikely that the blood tests for IgE will
be positive and they cannot provide you a definitive diagnosis.

Non-Gluten Wheat Allergies and Intolerances

Up to this point, we have discussed only gluten as an offensive
component of wheat. However, it is only one of many proteins
founds in wheat and its close relatives.

Gluten seems to be responsible for most reactions to wheat.
It is also possible to have an allergic reaction to wheat without
gluten being involved. These types of reactions to wheat are far
less common than the problems discussed in previous chapters.
Few people have this type of allergy to wheat, and even fewer
experience an anaphylactic reaction. But it is worth noting that
these reactions do exist.

In such cases the other gluten grains can usually be eaten.
However, it should be pointed out that spelt is extremely closely
related to wheat and may not be an acceptable alternative.

With a non-gluten reaction to wheat, all gliadin, gluten, and
celiac testing will be negative. But tests that measure your reaction
to whole wheat (rather than only to gluten) will be positive. If it is
a traditional allergy, as described above, skin testing for a wheat
allergy may be positive and the IgE blood test will also be positive.

But not all non-gluten reactions to wheat are of the traditional allergic variety. It is also possible to have a non-gluten reaction to wheat that is not an IgE antibody reaction, but more akin to a gluten intolerance, the difference being that it does not involve gluten. In this case, either the IgA or IgG antibody for wheat will be positive, and all reactions against gluten (gliadin) will be negative. IgE reactions to wheat will also be negative. The following results indicate a non-gluten intolerance to wheat, but not a gluten intolerance.

IgG and IgA gliadin antibody — negative

IgE wheat antibody — negative

IgG wheat antibody — positive

This is not a traditional wheat allergy. It is really a chronic wheat allergy, equivalent to a gluten intolerance but due to another component in the wheat. That component may or may not also be found in the close wheat relatives — rye, barley, spelt, and so on. Testing for antibody reactions to each of these foods is the best way to find out if they too cause a problem. An example of the type of testing that looks at reactions to wheat, barley, rye, gluten, and gliadin can be found in Appendix G.

It is fairly unusual to find IgG antibodies against one of these grains without also finding gliadin antibodies, but it does happen on occasion. Such results mean that the patient has an intolerance against that grain, but not a gluten intolerance. Some component of the grain other than gluten (gliadin) is the problem.

Hannah

For the past several years, Hannah has experienced chronic sinus problems, which she thought might be due to airborne allergies. She knew she should see the doctor about them, but she's so busy with her job as a bank manager and with her three children that she just didn't get around to it.

Then she started experiencing digestive upsets, including frequent gas, bloating, and cramps. While she could cope with the sinus discomfort and her runny nose, these new problems caused her both pain and embarrassment, interfering with her work and home life. So she finally made an appointment to see her doctor, who asked her to keep a food diary for a few weeks.

Suspecting that her symptoms might be related to wheat, the doctor had her tested for gluten intolerance. The test came back negative. Nevertheless, Hannah was desperate for relief and decided to try eliminating wheat from her diet. Her symptoms improved.

Hannah is fortunate to have a doctor who takes her patients' experience seriously. Because Hannah felt so much better when she stopped eating wheat, her doctor sent her to an allergist to be tested for a wheat allergy. Although the skin test was negative, a subsequent blood test showed that Hannah's body did produce IgG antibodies when exposed to wheat. While Hannah doesn't have a conventional IgE allergy to wheat or an intolerance to gluten, she does indeed have a wheat intolerance.

Summary

While much less common than gluten intolerance, other reactions to gluten, wheat, and other gluten-containing grains do exist. These include allergic reactions to inhaled wheat or gluten, allergic reactions to wheat or gluten applied to the skin, anaphylactic reactions to wheat or gluten, and allergic reactions to grain components other than gluten. These problems may be diagnosed through skin testing, in the case of conventional IgE allergies, or through blood testing for IgE or IgG antibodies.

part IV

Testing Summary for All Forms of Gluten Intolerance and Wheat Allergies

CHAPTER 7

Testing for Reactions to Wheat and Gluten

You cannot see anything that you do not first contemplate as a reality.

—Ramtha

When you suspect that wheat or gluten is causing you a problem, it is logical to want to be tested. Testing was covered in great detail in previous chapters. In this chapter, we present a summary of that information.

Who Should Be Tested?

Ideally everyone should be tested. If we were serious about providing the highest quality care possible and delivering true preventative medicine, then everyone would be screened as a child. Gluten intolerance is as common as or more common than many other conditions that our healthcare system routinely screens for, but most people are never tested, and it seems unlikely that this testing will become routine any time soon. This is even more unfortunate when you consider the number of other health problems that routine testing could prevent. Therefore, you have to take it upon yourself to make sure that you get tested.

For any kind of medical testing, it is important that you always get a copy of your lab work. There is no central repository for lab results, so you must take charge and keep lab records on your own. That way you'll never have to worry about trying to track them down later. If you aren't automatically given a copy of your results — which I encourage every practitioner to do — contact your clinic and request a copy.

Elimination Diets

One potential way to determine whether or not you are reacting to gluten is simply to eliminate it from your diet. But eliminating gluten is much easier said than done. You may try to avoid gluten but perhaps you don't successfully eliminate it entirely. Or you may not avoid it long enough to get results. Or you may simply be suffering from symptoms that are subtle and difficult to detect. These issues can complicate your ability to figure out whether or not gluten is truly a problem for you. This can be true whether you have celiac disease or not.

But eliminating wheat or gluten from your diet can potentially provide a wealth of information. However, many physicians would disagree with this statement and argue that you shouldn't do this. If you don't test positive for celiac disease, then many doctors are unlikely to support a treatment plan that includes the avoidance of gluten. This comes from the misconception that celiac disease is the only meaningful form, or is the most serious form, of gluten intolerance. We've already established that clinical evidence does not support this view, nor does a more logical and scientific view of the current medical literature.

Doctors are also concerned that if you start avoiding gluten before they can test you then their tests will be rendered irrelevant. This is true. But if you've already figured out that gluten is a problem for you, then what difference will a lab result make? And if you haven't figured it out or if you want the proof of a test result, then you can start eating gluten again and get tested.

Fundamentally, many physicians seem to think that going without gluten in your diet is such a drastic step that you should never consider it except under professional guidance. This is, of course, absurd. You are in charge of your health, and you are the one who continuously experiences a wealth of feedback from your body about how you feel. Some of us are more in tune with our bodies than others, but thousands of people have figured out, all on their own, that they are much better off when they don't eat gluten.

Many physicians also seem to believe that you won't take the diet seriously without a diagnosis of celiac disease. This will always be a problem for people, whether they have celiac disease or non-celiac gluten intolerance. Some people will take the avoidance of gluten seriously and others will avoid it only casually, if at all. Of course, you should take it seriously. Unfortunately many physicians don't yet appreciate the seriousness of non-celiac gluten intolerance and they convey this, consciously or unconsciously, to their patients. If this is the case for you, it can make it even more difficult to convince yourself that you really do need to avoid gluten.

Alex and Jennifer

Alex and his sister Jennifer have both suffered from a variety of seemingly mild health problems since they were children. They were both very colicky babies. Jennifer often feels very tired and Alex still has the acne he thought would disappear after adolescence. And they are prone to on-again, off-again IBS-type digestive symptoms, which flared up on a recent trip they took to Italy for a family reunion.

Both of them have wondered if their stomach problems are related to what they eat. After a friend was diagnosed with food allergies, Jennifer decided that she would try eliminating foods from her diet to see if she could pinpoint any troublesome ones. She had read that gluten was a common source of trouble, so she started with that. After several weeks of following a gluten-free diet, she felt much better. For her, this was proof enough that her symptoms were caused by gluten and she decided to maintain her new way of eating.

Alex, on the other hand, has always preferred to see things in black and white. He wouldn't feel sure about what was going on unless he was tested. He consulted a specialist, who explained the testing procedure.

"First, we'll run gliadin IgA and gliadin IgG antibody tests to see if your body reacts to gliadin. At the same time, we need to run a total IgA test to make sure that your body isn't deficient in IgA. If it is, it will affect the gliadin IgA test results."

Alex wasn't IgA deficient, but the gliadin antibody tests came back positive, showing that he did indeed have some kind of gluten intolerance.

"We can stop the testing right here," the doctor told him. "We've found out enough to know that you should stop eating gluten."

But Alex was still curious about what kind of intolerance he had, so the doctor ordered a tissue transglutaminase IgA test. This too came back positive, indicating celiac disease. When the specialist described the biopsy procedure, Alex decided that he already had enough information.

"Given how my sister's health has improved now that she's not eating gluten and the results of the blood tests, I don't need to go through the biopsy for any more proof," he said.

Since Alex would be cutting wheat and other sources of gluten out of his diet, the specialist also didn't think it was necessary to run tests for wheat allergies or an IgE gluten allergy.

Alex and Jennifer have helped each other adapt to their conditions. They took a course in gluten-free cooking and *have eliminated all gluten from their diets. They are both feeling better than they have for years.*

Lab Tests

While some people figure out that they are gluten intolerant by eliminating gluten from their diet, many prefer to see some lab work before they undertake such a venture. As we've discussed, in most cases blood tests can be used to determine whether or not you are reactive to wheat or gluten. Unfortunately, getting the proper lab testing done can be very difficult. In addition, as we have also pointed out, testing is not perfect and doesn't necessarily correlate with the symptoms that a person is experiencing, which can vary significantly from one person to the next. That being said, blood tests are still excellent tools for determining whether or not you have a reaction to wheat or gluten. Blood tests and other testing were discussed more fully in Chapters 4 and 5. Here we will summarize their use and try to prioritize them.

Most physicians have several choices of tests available to them: gliadin IgA, gliadin IgG, tissue transglutaminase IgA, reticulin IgA, and endomysial IgA antibody tests. Some physicians select a *panel* that includes all of these. Others select various components based on habit or preference.

Ideally, you should have both of the gliadin tests and the tissue transglutaminase IgA test, along with a total IgA test. While it is fairly common for physicians to run the gliadin tests and the tissue transglutaminase IgA test, the most common error is not running a total IgA test with them. Without it they can't determine whether or not you are IgA deficient. This is important because if you are, then the results of the other IgA tests may be falsely negative.

The next most common mistake is for physicians to ignore the gliadin antibody test results. Because these tests do not indicate whether or not someone has celiac disease, positive results are interpreted as only suggesting the need for further testing for celiac disease. In fact, one has to wonder why these tests are run at all, since historically they haven't been considered diagnostic for anything. But researchers have known for a long time that gliadin antibodies provide useful information, which is why the gliadin testing gets run. Fortunately the gliadin antibody tests *are* commonly run and, properly interpreted, they tell us a great deal.

The following flow diagrams prioritize the tests used in the diagnosis of gluten intolerance and wheat allergies through blood tests. These diagrams are not meant to provide any detailed information on these tests or the reasoning behind them. They are designed solely to help you put together all of the information presented up to this point in the book.

The first diagram provides a simple explanation of the types of testing readily available to most physicians. It also gives you an idea about how these tests relate to each other. The second diagram covers testing for reactions to wheat that may or may not include gluten intolerance, as well as IgE allergy testing for gliadin. These tests are less common and require seeing a specialist in food allergies and intolerances.

This chapter is merely a short summary to help you prioritize testing and understand how the tests relate to each other. This can be confusing because it is a complex subject. You should refer back to Chapters 4, 5, and 6 for more details on these tests and why they were selected. It is important to understand the material covered in those chapters in order to understand testing for wheat allergies, celiac disease, and non-celiac forms of gluten intolerance.

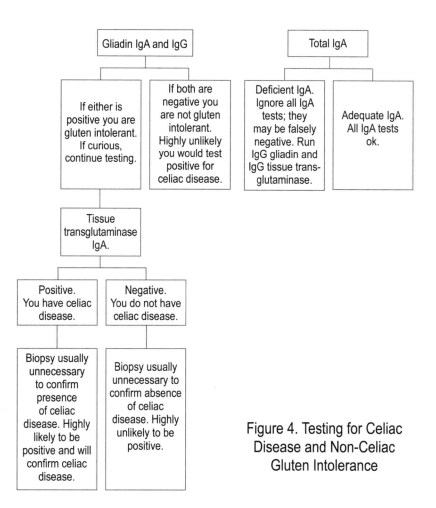

Figure 4. Testing for Celiac Disease and Non-Celiac Gluten Intolerance

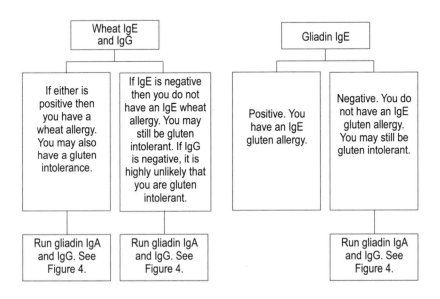

Figure 5. Testing for Wheat Allergy and Gluten Allergy
Note: Skin testing may also be helpful for diagnosing IgE wheat and gluten allergies.

CHAPTER 8

Infants, Children, and Gluten Intolerance

We cannot direct the wind,
but we can adjust the sails.

—Bertha Calloway, founder of the
Great Plains Black Museum

Gluten intolerance is just as common in infants and children as it is in adults, and, as with adults, it can have serious consequences. If we tested more infants and children for gluten intolerance, we would likely prevent most cases of celiac disease as well as many other problems. Unfortunately testing often doesn't happen until they are very ill. All of the issues regarding testing discussed in Chapters 4 and 5, except as discussed in this chapter, are the same for infants and children as they are for adults.

Infants

Infants, even those who are only breast-feeding, can suffer from a gluten intolerance. Some of their symptoms are different from those of adults. And of course, they can't communicate their discomfort to us verbally. Here are some of the more common symptoms seen in infants:

+ Crying more than average
+ Colic
+ Poor sleep
+ Very foul stools

+ Constipation
+ Bad gas
+ Spitting up or burping a lot
+ Eczema
+ Failure to thrive
+ Just plain orneriness

As with adults, infants who are gluten intolerant may not have any noticeable symptoms.

The Role of Breast-Feeding

Breast-feeding infants can be subject to a gluten problem in two different ways. First, they may be born with a gluten intolerance. When they ingest components of gluten from their mothers' breast milk, they react to it like any other gluten intolerant person. Their immune system detects the gluten and forms an immune reaction against it, producing gliadin antibodies as discussed in detail earlier in this book.

The second way is unique to infants. It is well accepted now that breast-feeding is very good for infants for a variety of reasons. One of these reasons is that breast milk helps to protect the infant by giving him or her a stronger immune system. As part of this protection, breast-feeding infants ingest their mothers' antibodies, found in her breast milk. However, if the mother has a gluten intolerance and continues to eat gluten, then she is making antibodies against gluten, which she passes on to her infant in her breast milk. These antibodies can then trigger in the infant an inflammatory immune response against gluten. In this case the infant may not have been born with a gluten intolerance, but its immune system is obliged to respond to the antibodies in the breast milk. Antibodies are essentially flags. A problem — in this case gluten — is being flagged.

Therefore the infant's immune system will respond, even though the infant did not produce the antibodies.

For this reason, when treating breast-feeding infants it is very important to evaluate the mother for gluten intolerance (as well as for an intolerance or allergy to other foods). If she is gluten intolerant, then removing gluten from her diet is an important part of treating the infant. However, even if she isn't gluten intolerant, if the *infant* is gluten intolerant the mother still needs to avoid gluten during the period that she is breast-feeding her infant.

There have been several studies on the impact of breast-feeding on the development of celiac disease. These studies have not looked at non-celiac forms of gluten intolerance, but they may shed light on this issue as well. Breast-feeding has not been shown to prevent celiac disease. However, breast-feeding seems to delay its onset. This is especially true if an infant continues to breast-feed for at least two months after gluten is introduced into its diet. These studies have also found that when gluten is introduced at either too early or too late an age, this benefit is lost. In addition, introducing large amounts of gluten at weaning is associated with an increase in the risk of developing celiac disease.

The current best recommendation, based on the research available, is to introduce gluten between four and six months of age while still breast-feeding the infant. It is also recommended that gluten be introduced gradually and only in small amounts. However, if you are very suspicious that your child will be gluten intolerant, then it may be wise to delay the introduction of gluten for as long as possible, at least one to two years and maybe indefinitely. There is no reason that you *must* introduce gluten into your child's diet. And, even if you are breast-feeding when you do so, it will not prevent the inevitable.

Testing Infants

Infants *can* be tested for gluten intolerance. The blood tests for antibodies to gliadin, wheat, barley, rye, and other foods, discussed in Chapter 5, are just as relevant for infants as they are for adults. But testing specifically for celiac disease often returns negative results because infants have not yet had time to develop villous atrophy.

When testing for any antibodies in breast-fed infants, it is important to be aware of the possibility that the antibodies may not actually belong to the infant. They may be coming from the mother's breast milk. As discussed above, this is why the mother should be tested as well. If a breast-feeding infant does test positive for these antibodies and the mother is found to be gluten intolerant and is still ingesting gluten, then the child may be retested at a later age to determine whether the antibodies originated from the mother or the infant. Retesting is required only if gluten is reintroduced into the child's diet. If the infant did not have a gluten intolerance but was reacting to the mother's gluten intolerance via her antibodies, it may be possible to safely reintroduce gluten into the child's diet.

Although testing can be done at a very young age, in practice it is usually avoided because it is usually very easy to control the infant's diet and, therefore, easy to remove gluten on a trial basis. Testing should focus first on the mother and, if it shows that she is positive for gluten intolerance, then she should of course remove gluten from her diet. She can also do a trial elimination of gluten from her diet. If this satisfactorily improves the health of the infant then the goal has been achieved, at least temporarily.

Children

Gluten intolerance in children can potentially cause most of the symptoms listed for adults in Chapter 3. However, out of this long list of problems, children are more likely to experience one or more of the following:

+ Digestive problems
+ Abdominal pain
+ Headaches
+ Chronic ear infections
+ Fatigue
+ Eczema
+ Poor growth

Some of the problems seen in adults are much less likely to be seen in children because they do not develop until a later age. This is certainly true of most of the autoimmune conditions associated with gluten intolerance, though not all, such as juvenile rheumatoid arthritis. And osteoporosis is also not diagnosed until much later in life, although childhood is the most important time for establishing the foundation for strong bones. Also, gluten intolerant children are not often anemic, but they can exhibit low iron stores, indicating that they are not absorbing iron well and may eventually become anemic.

It is a misconception that children can outgrow a food intolerance or allergy. While it may appear to happen, what is really occurring in most of these cases is that the children are outgrowing their symptoms. For example, they may have nausea or vomiting when they are young, but not when they're older. Or for a few years they may have chronic ear infections. Later on they develop different — seemingly unrelated — symptoms that are in fact also due to their gluten intolerance. Maybe they have head-aches or diarrhea or constipation or any of the other problems we've noted earlier in this book.

The child did not outgrow the gluten intolerance. The intol-erance is still there, but as the body changes, the symptoms can change. This isn't well understood yet, but frequently, for whatever reason, the problem is pushed to a different part of the body or a different weakness develops, and the inflammation that is being triggered becomes most noticeable there. The common thread is that all of these symptoms are related either to inflammation (which is triggered by the immune response to gluten) or to the malabsorption of nutrients.

Celiac Disease in Children

Children are just as susceptible to celiac disease as adults. However, because the antibody levels and villous atrophy necessary to detect it can take a while to develop, testing children for celiac disease before the age of two is considered relatively inaccurate. However, this should not prevent you from testing for non-celiac gluten intol-erance. For either type of testing, the age at which it is useful will vary depending on when gluten is introduced into the diet.

Even a child with a strong family history of celiac disease may not test positive for it for many years. However, if celiac disease is strongly suspected in a child due to family history or siblings with celiac disease, it is wise not to wait for it to develop. Testing for non-celiac forms of gluten intolerance will indicate whether or not gluten is a problem for this child. If those tests are posi-tive, the child should avoid gluten, which will prevent the possible development of celiac disease.

Testing Children for Non-Celiac Gluten Intolerance

The procedure for testing for gliadin antibodies and for the antibodies against wheat, barley, rye, and other foods is the same for children as it is for adults, as discussed in Chapter 5. Typically, positive results will show up on blood tests within months of introducing gluten into the diet. Catching this problem at as early an age as possible can prevent many years of suffering and poor health.

Tyler

Tyler was a colicky baby, but he got worse when solid foods were introduced. From the very first time Tyler was fed solids he had trouble keeping food down. As he grew older, he suffered from alternating constipation and diarrhea, stomach pains, rashes, and constant coughing. These symptoms affected him daily, turning a once reasonably happy baby into an unhappy and uncomfortable little boy.

For years, his frustrated parents, searching for a way to help their son, took him from doctor to doctor. He was diagnosed with everything from asthma to encopresis (resistance to bowel movements). However, none of these diagnoses or their treatments seemed to get at the root of Tyler's problems, which continued to have a negative impact on his quality of life every day.

When Tyler was 6 years old, his parents took him to a doctor specializing in food intolerances and allergies. When he was tested for gluten intolerance, they finally had the answer they'd been looking for. While removing gluten from Tyler's diet was a challenge at first, he and his family soon adapted and now, at the age of 8, he is symptom free, active, and happy.

Summary

Infants and children can suffer from celiac disease and non-celiac forms of gluten intolerance. They may exhibit a number of symptoms or none at all. The conditions associated with gluten intolerance can cause serious health issues both in childhood and later in life.

Most of the benefits of early detection should be obvious by now. But it is still important to emphasize that the sooner gluten intolerance is discovered, the better. Infants or children whose intolerance is found early will be much healthier and are likely to continue to be healthier throughout life. They will absorb nutrients better and will be much closer to optimal health than they would have been otherwise. Studies have also shown that once gluten is removed from the diet, children who have suffered from poor growth tend to catch up. And the younger the child is at diagnosis, the better the chance that he or she will catch up. Long term health starts in infancy and continues throughout our lives. There should be no doubt that the earlier a gluten intolerance is discovered, the better off a person will be.

part V

Treating Gluten Intolerance

CHAPTER 9

Treating Gluten Intolerance and Wheat/Gluten Allergies

Education is when you read the fine print.
Experience is what you get if you don't.
— Pete Seeger (b. 1919), singer and composer

An ounce of prevention is worth a pound of cure.
— Attributed to Henry de Bracton (c. 1210–1268),
English jurist, and to Benjamin Franklin (1706–1790)

If you are intolerant or allergic to wheat or gluten, the only way to truly solve your problem is to avoid them. There are no shortcuts to treating a gluten intolerance or allergy. Complete avoidance is the only way to truly optimize your health. Many companies and individuals have made claims about products and treatments that can solve this problem without eliminating gluten from your diet, but none has stood up to rigorous investigation. First we will discuss the avoidance of gluten, and then we will focus on wheat.

Celiac disease provides an excellent example on how to resolve problems caused by a gluten intolerance. We know that essentially no amount of gluten is acceptable in the diet of someone who is celiac. The same is true for those with non-celiac forms of gluten intolerance, unless of course you feel that doing some damage to your body is acceptable. While eliminating gluten is much easier said than done, tens of thousands of people successfully follow a strict gluten-free diet. If they can do it, then you can, too. Also in your favor is the growing market for gluten-free products, which has inspired the development of new products for those of us who don't eat gluten, making it easier today to avoid gluten than at any other time in recent memory.

There has been some debate on the definition of *gluten free*. This term is applied primarily to processed foods, but can also be applied to any food that might normally come into contact with even a minute amount of gluten. The Gluten-Free Certification Organization (www.GFCO.org), a program run by the Gluten Intolerance Group of North America, certifies only those foods that have less than 10 parts per million (ppm) gluten. This is well below the standard suggested by research studies that indicate that the maximum allowable amount of gluten for someone suffering from celiac disease is somewhere between 20 and 200 ppm.

Avoiding Gluten

Gluten, as we noted earlier, is a protein found in wheat, rye, barley, and a number of other grains, as well as in hundreds of products produced from these grains. The following is a list of base grains and grain-like products that should be avoided.

✦ Wheat	✦ Bulgur
✦ Spelt	✦ Wheat germ
✦ Rye	✦ Couscous
✦ Barley	✦ Farina
✦ Kamut	✦ Emmer
✦ Durum	✦ Matzoh
✦ Triticale	✦ Graham
✦ Einkorn	✦ Sprouted wheat
✦ Semolina	

You need to know this list so that you can read labels and effectively avoid gluten. Although it may seem overwhelming as the significance of a gluten intolerance starts to sink in, keep in mind that millions of people on this planet don't eat gluten and that there are many gluten-free products available.

Breads

Gluten is the ingredient in bread that makes it springy and stretchy. It allows bread to be light and fluffy without being crumbly. Because gluten is a component of all of the grains listed above, it is in nearly all bread products including wheat bread, white bread, rye bread, sourdough bread, and flour tortillas, as well as most kinds of rolls, muffins, cookies, cakes, and pie crusts, since they are all made out of these grains. So are pancakes, waffles, hamburger buns, hot dog buns, croutons, and most crackers. Fortunately, a number of companies are producing a variety of gluten-free bread products. Many of these are listed in Appendix C.

Battered, Breaded, and Deep-Fried Foods

Batters and breadings made with flour almost certainly contain gluten. Flour is simply ground grain and you can assume that these coatings are made with wheat flour. Onion rings, chicken strips, fish sticks, deep-fried cheese sticks, the fish in fish and chips, and many other deep-fried items are breaded and therefore contain gluten. Breaded or battered foods may also be baked rather than deep-fried.

It should be pointed out here that if the same oil is used to deep fry a breaded food and something non-breaded, such as French fries, then the non-breaded food can become contaminated with gluten. Also, sometimes foods are prepared with a flour mixture that you aren't aware of. For example, French fries are sometimes rolled in a spice/flour mix.

Pasta

Pasta is made from flour. Therefore, all pasta can be assumed to contain gluten, regardless of its size or shape. This is true for semolina, durum, and spinach pastas too.

However, a wide variety of fine gluten-free pasta alternatives are available now. They are typically made from rice flour or corn flour, but others also exist. Many of these are listed in Appendix C.

Beer

All beer contains barley and therefore contains gluten. This includes ale, lager, and stout. Believe it or not, there are some new gluten-free beer alternatives that actually taste like beer. Bard's Tale and Red Bridge are two.

Barley Malt

Barley malt is, of course, made from barley. Sometimes listed only as malt, it is an inexpensive sweetener often used in cereals and other processed foods. Be sure to look for it when reading ingredients.

Flour and Gluten as an Additive

Flour is frequently added to processed foods. In particular, soups, sauces, gravies, and spice mixes often contain some form of gluten. Even salad dressing can have gluten in it. Anything that is processed, whether it comes in a can, jar, or any other kind of packaging, can potentially contain gluten. You must read all ingredients.

Soy Sauce

Soy sauce is made from two primary ingredients, soy and wheat. It deserves special attention because it is used so widely. Fortunately, tamari, a soy sauce that is often wheat free, is available. However, not all tamari is wheat free. You must double-check.

Deli Meats

Deli meats may be coated with flour or injected with something that contains gluten. You should check the ingredients with the manufacturer. Fortunately, some deli meat manufacturers are now promoting the fact that they are gluten free, making it easier to determine which products are safe.

Play-Doh

Yes, even Play-Doh contains wheat. Unfortunately, young children sometimes like to taste their Play-Doh creations. However, gluten-free alternatives are available or you can make your own. Sources and recipes can be found online.

Medications and Supplements

Some medications and supplements contain gluten. Supplements include vitamins, minerals, and other non-prescription items such as botanical medicines and amino acids. Supplement labels, surprisingly enough, are more likely to provide a complete list of ingredients than are the labels on prescription and over-the-counter medications. If all the ingredients aren't listed on the packaging or paperwork that comes with your medication, then ask your pharmacist or look it up yourself. You may want to contact the company or look online for information about the medication and its inactive ingredients.

Foods Deserving Special Consideration

Oats

The question of whether or not oats contain gluten has been the source of considerable confusion over the years. It turns out that oats do not contain gluten. However, they can potentially be contaminated with a fairly significant amount of gluten. This contamination is the result of the fact that oats are often handled by or stored in the same mills, processing equipment, train cars, and grain elevators that handle wheat, barley, and rye.

Gluten free oats are available from Bob's Red Mill (though not all of their oat probucts are gluten free), Cream Hill Estates (www.creamhillestates.com), Gifts of Nature (www.giftsofnature.net), Gluten Free Oats (www.glutenfreeoats.com), and Only Oats (www.onlyoats.ca). These companies (also listed in Appendix C) take special care to avoid cross-contamination and to produce truly gluten-free oats. Any reaction to gluten-free oats is simply a reaction to oats, not to gluten.

Buckwheat

Buckwheat sounds like it would be a source of gluten. However, it is a very distant relative of wheat (see Figure 2 in Chapter 2) and does not contain gluten. It is perfectly acceptable in a gluten-free diet.

Caramel Coloring

Caramel coloring can be produced from a variety of sources, including gluten-containing grains. However, in the United States and Canada, all reports indicate that manufacturers have not been using gluten in the production of their caramel. This may not be true of all countries.

Modified Food Starch

Like caramel, modified food starch can be produced from a variety of sources, including gluten grains. Fortunately, in the United States and Canada, all reports state that modified food starch does not contain gluten. This may not be true in other countries.

Corn Gluten

Corn gluten is completely different from the gluten that is being addressed in this book. Corn, corn gluten, and anything derived from corn are acceptable parts of a gluten-free diet.

Blue Cheese

Blue cheese acquires its characteristic blue veins from a mold introduced during the cheese-making process to create the environment necessary for making blue cheese. Originally, this mold came from moldy bread, which was ground up and added to the cheese. Nowadays the mold is typically acquired from more standardized sources and does not contain gluten. In most cases, then, blue cheese is safe for those avoiding gluten. However, it is still possible to find blue cheese made with bread mold, so you should check with the manufacturer just to be safe.

Vinegar

Vinegar has been another source of confusion. Vinegar can be made from many different foods, including wine, apple cider, grapes (balsamic), and grains such as wheat. White vinegar is usually made from a gluten grain, but it is also usually distilled, which removes any gluten. Distilled vinegar is gluten free. Malt vinegar is not distilled and is not gluten free.

Distilled Alcohol and Spirits

Distilled alcohol and spirits are also gluten free. These include whiskey, scotch, vodka, tequila (which never had gluten in it to begin with), brandy, and gin. However, whiskey and liquors may have coloring or other additives that are added after the distillation process and should be carefully evaluated.

Processed Foods

Remember, any processed food product may contain gluten. *You must read the list of ingredients on all packages.* Be aware of the possibility that even if gluten is not listed, the food may still be contaminated due to processing techniques shared with other foods or due to flour used in the handling of the food.

The safest processed foods are certified gluten free. On the product label look for "GF" with a circle around it. Companies using this symbol have met strict production standards, have had their product tested for gluten, and must pass regular on-site inspections. Some companies are coming up with their own symbols, but they have not necessarily met the same criteria. Visit the Gluten Free Certification Organization at www. gfco.org for more information about this program.

Dining Out

Dining out can be challenging, but there are usually options on the menu which are acceptable or can be prepared gluten free with relatively minor changes. Unfortunately, there is still the issue of contamination to consider. But fortunately there are many restaurants taking special steps to meet the needs of those who are gluten intolerant. In fact, you may be surprised to discover that many local eateries and national chains are already catering to the gluten-free crowd. Many of these restaurants are members of the Gluten Free Restaurant Awareness Program® (GFRAP). Members of this program take a special interest in understanding and serving those who must avoid gluten. More information about this program and the restaurants participating in it is available at www.glutenfreerestaurants.org.

Avoiding Wheat

As we've discussed, most people who react to wheat are also reacting to gluten; therefore, they need to avoid all of the gluten-containing grains and products. But if you only need to avoid wheat then the list of offending foods is slightly shorter.

Wheat includes triticale, semolina, kamut, and couscous. Spelt, although a different grain, is an extremely close genetic relative of wheat and may not be acceptable for those who cannot tolerate wheat. Little research has been done on this issue, so proceed cautiously. Barley and rye, both gluten-containing grains, are acceptable options for those avoiding only wheat. And all of the non-gluten grains are also acceptable wheat free alternatives.

Contamination of Gluten-Free Foods

What if a gluten-free food is made in a factory that also handles gluten? This is a common question. Ideally you should avoid it. But the next question is "How much gluten can contaminated food have?" The answer depends on many aspects of the factory and its processing. Did the potato chip run immediately follow a run of a gluten-containing food, or did they use the same oil? Is the factory the size of a football field, with the gluten-containing products at one end and the gluten-free ones at the other, or is the gluten-free line right next to the gluten-containing line? How clean is the facility?

Unfortunately, it can be very difficult to know the answers to these questions, and even if you do, the answer still may not be black or white because the problems potentially caused by contamination can also depend on how sensitive your body is to detecting gluten in your food. Some people can tell when there is unlisted gluten contamination in their food. Others have no idea.

Of course, this question also involves the quality of your diet. If you eat a lot of processed food, then you're more likely to run into contamination. If you eat processed food only occasionally, then it's far less likely to be a problem for you.

During the first few weeks and months of your gluten-free diet, you should not worry too much about this type of contamination. You have much bigger fish to fry. You are making such a large change in your diet that you will experience dramatic benefits and will unlikely be able to detect differences caused by very small amounts of contamination, although some people still can. However, as you become more skilled at following a gluten-free diet and as your body gets used to the idea of feeling good again, it may be worth the effort to work on avoiding these potential gluten intrusions.

Contamination can also occur right in your own kitchen. Home is often where the gluten is. If other family members are eating regular bread and other gluten-containing foods, then you'll want to be sure that your food is not contaminated by their food. You should always use clean plates, bowls, cups, silverware, and mixing utensils. Also use clean pots and pans when you prepare your food. Some people go so far as to have completely separate kitchenware, but this is not required. However, you may need to have separate butter dishes and jars of peanut butter, jam, and mayonnaise. Just look at these products after they've been used and you'll often see little bread crumbs.

The big question is the toaster. Do you really need a separate toaster? While most crumbs fall to the bottom of the toaster, it is certainly possible for a toaster to contaminate your gluten-free bread. If this is an issue in your household, then you should get a separate toaster. A toaster is a very useful product for a gluten-free diet, since most gluten-free breads hold together better and taste better after being toasted.

How Much Gluten Is Too Much?

It is generally agreed that people with celiac disease should completely avoid gluten. However, how seriously people with other forms of gluten intolerance must take their gluten avoidance is often questioned. Why is this?

We base these ideas on how severe we think the potential consequences of eating gluten might be, not on the potential benefits of avoiding gluten. For example, when someone has a life-threatening allergy to peanuts, we recommend that they never touch even the smallest amount of peanut. This is the prudent thing to do. With celiac disease, we know that even though it isn't as life-threatening as a peanut allergy, in order to heal and stay healthy, one must avoid all sources of gluten.

Consider smoking. Is one cigarette a day okay? How about one a month? Is second-hand smoke okay? Or does exposure even in these small quantities have the potential to cause significant health problems? And will completely avoiding it be better for you in the long run? We know that there are potential health consequences of even the occasional cigarette, or simply inhaling second-hand smoke. We also know that if you've smoked for many years, the potential health consequences of smoking greatly increase. So either way, you are much better off if you don't smoke.

Or consider a virus, something more akin to a reaction to gluten. If your immune system constantly has to try to rid itself of a virus, this taxes the body. And the greater the viral load, the harder it must work. Herpes zoster (shingles) is an excellent example. If you have this virus then it is always in your body, but it produces noticeable symptoms only when you are stressed or your immune system is challenged. Then your immune system can no longer keep it in check.

The same is true for the ingestion of gluten. If you have a non-celiac form of gluten intolerance and you have been eating gluten for many years, you've accumulated a history of ingesting something that is toxic to your body. You may notice that avoiding it 95% of the time relieves the symptom that you are treating, but you are still suffering some ill effects of ingesting gluten, whether you realize it or not. And it takes energy for your body to continuously deal with the problem (gluten). It also increases the load on your immune system and decreases its ability to deal with other problems.

The point here is that the more thorough you are at avoiding gluten, the healthier you'll be. If you want to truly optimize your health, you should avoid all sources of gluten. Of course, the choice is yours. But remember that the symptoms you experience from ingesting gluten are not the same as the damage that is being caused. Even if you perceive no symptoms at all, your body may still be undergoing damage.

Coping with the Transition to a Gluten-Free Diet

Withdrawal Symptoms

When first eliminating gluten from their diets, some people go through what can best be described as withdrawal symptoms. In these cases, breaking away from wheat and gluten is more profound than they thought. They may crave gluten terribly for the first few days or weeks. They may get headaches or fatigue or just feel crummy. If this happens to you, hang in there. You'll get over it and things will get better.

The Social Impact

One the most challenging issues is "How do I cope with the social impact of having a food allergy?" Most everyone else will be eating gluten just about everywhere you go, although after you go gluten free you may be surprised to learn about others doing the same thing. But not everyone will be supportive. Regardless, how you handle it will depend a lot on your personality and your relationships. And whether you want to or not, you are going to learn a lot about yourself and those around you.

You may want to talk to your friends and family about your food allergies and about how they can support you. Some people are very open and have no problem informing those around them. That is probably the healthiest approach. If you are strong about your convictions, others will likely follow your lead. But regardless of how comfortable you are with this approach, educating those around you about the negative health impact that gluten has on you is really all that you can do. Then if they are interested in learning more you can begin to fill them in.

If you are sincere and forthright about your situation then you certainly can't hold yourself responsible for how other people perceive you. Some will be very supportive, some will do nothing, and others will take it as a personal offense to their hospitality. Responses from family and friends may vary widely. In some families, everyone will join in the gluten-free diet. In others, gluten-intolerant family members have separate foods. Some friends will go out of their way to accommodate your needs. Others just won't understand. But even when people want to be helpful they often don't really understand the issue or its significance well enough to always provide you with gluten-free food. The bottom line is that it's *your* issue, not theirs. Learn how to take care of yourself and don't expect others to do it for you.

Some people don't bring it up at all in social situations, preferring to deal with it behind the scenes — eating before a social occasion, ordering things they know will be safe, or making sure they have something with them that they can eat. Different situations may call for different approaches. When going to someone's house for dinner, you may want to speak to your hosts ahead of time, or you may choose to eat before the party. If they aren't particularly understanding at first, hopefully they will eventually come around. At a restaurant, you may feel comfortable asking your waiter about the food. If not, you might phone ahead of time or order only foods you know are safe.

Remember, you are a leader in a growing and important field. If you are the first in your circle to introduce this issue of gluten intolerance, others will likely benefit from your experience in the future. The interest in this field is growing rapidly, as are the numbers of people discovering that they are better off without gluten.

Don't Stress Out

At times it may be tempting to break down and cry, but remind yourself that you've actually found a solution to your problem.[12] You've spent your life poisoning yourself without realizing it. Now you can control your problem and reverse most, if not all, of the damage. Life will actually be much better.

---

12 If avoiding gluten does not solve your health problems, then there is another underlying cause that hasn't been found yet. This is addressed in Chapter 12.

You aren't going to figure out this diet overnight. It is a learning process and will take time. In fact, the learning will go on throughout your life. The Gluten Intolerance Group of North America (GIG) is an excellent resource, providing information, education, and a variety of programs that support those with all forms of gluten intolerance.

GIG's Stepwise Program

GIG has a useful stepwise program available on their website (www.gluten.net) to help you avoid gluten. It encourages you to attack the big sources of gluten first and to celebrate that accomplishment before moving on to more complex sources of gluten. What follows is a modified version of their concept.

Step 1: Eliminate the obvious sources of gluten from your diet: bread, pasta, beer, and cereal. The gluten in these foods likely makes up a huge percentage of the gluten in your diet, so this is an excellent start. Start looking for some of the gluten-free alternatives on the market. We'll discuss these shortly, but it won't take long to realize that many do exist!

Step 2: Once you feel comfortable with Step 1, start reading labels for hidden sources of gluten. This one will be a shocker, and you'll probably miss many sources of gluten in the early days of the learning process. You may want to make a list of the things you should avoid or refer back to this book. You may also want to make a list of the acceptable foods you find.

At this stage, it's also an excellent idea to have a gluten-free buddy whom you can talk to. You may be surprised to learn that a relative or co-worker avoids gluten or knows someone else who is gluten intolerant. Tap into the support network at GIG or one of the other agencies, or find a forum online. Many resources are listed in Appendix B.

Step 3: Fine tune your diet and begin to look at products like medicines, mouthwash, toothpaste, breath mints, and chewing gum. Consider cross-contamination issues such as shared foods and equipment in your kitchen.

Step 4: By this time you are probably quite adept at the diet. Do a little investigative research by contacting companies and asking them specifically about the ingredients in their foods. If you suspect there is something that isn't listed on the label or if you just want some peace of mind, then call them up.

If these steps seem overwhelming, stay at each one until you feel ready to go on.

Attitude Is Everything!

It is normal to go through the stages of loss — anger, denial, sadness — when making such a large change in your life. You are allowed that. But remember that you've got many options and you can make choices. No one wants to hear you complain about your condition. One energetic and positive woman who runs a support group for people who are gluten intolerant maintains a positive focus in her group, telling the members at the beginning of each meeting that there will be no whining about their loss. This may not be an acceptable strategy in the world of psychology, but her approach works. If you don't want to follow a gluten-free diet, then don't. You won't be the first person who didn't care enough about his or her health to make a positive change to improve it, and you certainly won't be the last. But hopefully you'll come around to the idea that it is worth doing.

Richard

Although he was happy to finally find out what was causing his health problems, Richard's heart sank when he was told it was a gluten intolerance. He and his wife, Claire, were overwhelmed with the prospect of adapting to the gluten-free diet that was the only treatment that could help him.

Richard's doctor had several suggestions to help them. He suggested that they first eliminate the largest sources of gluten in Richard's diet. Then they could focus on the less obvious sources. He also encouraged Richard to attend the meetings of a local support group.

Realizing that Richard must either accept this new way of eating or continue to damage his health, Claire and Richard immediately put the doctor's plan into action. Richard met many helpful people at the support group and, as he talked about his diagnosis with friends and family, he discovered that several people he knew suffered from a gluten intolerance. Through them, he learned about hidden sources of gluten, gluten-free alternatives, restaurants that were good for those on a gluten-free diet, and how to avoid contamination. Networking with other sufferers saved Claire and Richard time they would have spent researching, as well as helping them avoid many dietary errors.

They also decided that instead of taking a negative approach to this new diet, they would enjoy trying recipes and finding new things to eat. They both kept a notebook of safe foods and foods to avoid. And while Claire was free to eat gluten, she found that the attention she was now paying to Richard's diet paid off for her, too. As Richard eliminated gluten-containing foods from his diet, he replaced them with more nutritious alternatives. As a result, they were both eating a more healthy diet and they both felt better for it.

The Gluten-Free Diet

What Is Left to Eat?

When they first start a gluten-free diet, people often feel that there is nothing left to eat. But entire cultures — billions of people — thrive very nicely on diets with little or no gluten. In reality, what is left to eat is just about everything that is healthy for you. All vegetables, fruits, meats (except for some deli meats, as discussed above), rice, and beans still remain as viable and healthy options. Even dairy products are acceptable if you do not have a dairy allergy or intolerance, which is common in people who are gluten intolerant (see Chapter 12). The following foods do not contain gluten and can be included in a gluten-free diet:

- Soy
- Rice
- Corn
- Potatoes
- Beans
- Meats
- Fish
- Vegetables
- Fruits
- Nuts
- Dairy products
- Eggs
- Quinoa
- Millet
- Teff
- Tapioca
- Amaranth
- Arrowroot
- Buckwheat
- Montina

The Good News

The most challenging part of a gluten-free diet is finding processed or refined foods that are gluten free. If you haven't been eating a healthy diet, then you may need to get used to spending a little more time preparing your food. However, a benefit of the research into gluten intolerance and of the growing number of people avoiding gluten is that there are now many gluten-free breads, pastas, and other foods on the market, and new products are coming out all the time. You can get gluten-free cereals, cookies, cake mixes, brownie mixes, pancake mixes, bread mixes, and just about everything else under the sun. Interestingly, it's very possible to maintain a completely gluten-free diet and still eat primarily junk food. In fact, some people do just that. You don't want to do that, but you might want the occasional treat.

Gluten-free foods can often be found in local health-food stores and, more recently, at major chain grocers, especially places such as Whole Foods and Wild Oats. Products are also available online at the many gluten-free food retailers (see Appendix C for a list of some of these).

There are many excellent books on living gluten free, including cookbooks, and they are far more detailed than this chapter. It is not the intent of this book to reproduce the work of these fine authors. See Appendix B for a list of recommended reading and other resources for going gluten free.

But It's More Expensive to Eat Gluten Free!

If you insist on eating processed and refined carbohydrates, then yes, it is more expensive. But if you eat the healthy foods listed above, it's not. You have the choice. You don't have to buy expensive gluten-free products. You can be healthy and happy without them.

The reason that gluten-free foods are expensive is twofold. One is that they are produced in much smaller quantities; therefore they are more expensive to make. The second is that the gluten-containing options are designed to be cheap. The food industry is a gigantic business that uses products such as wheat, corn syrup, and cane sugar that are produced by the trainload. This gives you the impression that you are getting food for very little money. What you are really getting is often a stripped-down version of a whole food, something that now barely qualifies as food and has little nutritional value, which is why it has a very low price. The processed food industry has little to do with nutrition. It's mostly about marketing, branding, and convincing people that they can't live without something they'd certainly be better off without.

The healthiest gluten-free foods — "whole foods" such as vegetables, fruits, meats, nuts, and so on — are not special products and are still the same price that they were when you ate gluten. Look for them on the perimeter of the grocery store.

Will I Outgrow It?

There is no evidence that a gluten intolerance will go away. It's not like a virus or a bacteria that you can kill off. If you keep eating gluten, then you keep triggering your immune system to react to it. And the damage it causes can never fully heal, because you keep reintroducing the problem into your body.

You don't outgrow a gluten intolerance, although it may seem like it because your symptoms may change during your life. Your gluten intolerance may not always cause you to feel the same way, but the immune response is still there. As long as you continue to eat gluten, the lab results will stay the same or potentially get worse.

After you've avoided gluten for a while, the antibody levels that indicated your gluten intolerance will begin to decrease and in most cases eventually you will test negative for gluten intolerance. This does *not* mean that you are cured. Your antibody levels went down because you avoided the food to which your immune system was reacting. But your immune system has memory cells that remember your gluten intolerance, and if you start eating gluten again, your antibody levels will start to rise.

Don't fool yourself into thinking that you are cured if you reintroduce gluten and it doesn't seem to bother you anymore.

Some people have a dramatic reaction if they try to reintroduce it; others don't notice anything, even if they have had a dramatic reaction in the past. After eating gluten for several weeks or months, you will get sick again, although your health may degrade so gradually that you do not associate it with gluten. Some people do this after forgetting that they had a gluten intolerance and wonder why they don't feel well anymore.

How Long Will It Take to Heal?

It may take several weeks or months of a gluten-free diet before you begin to notice a difference in your health. Do not be disappointed if your problem isn't solved within a week or two. The healing process takes several months or even years, depending on your age and how long you've had the problem. Research on celiac disease has clearly shown that it can take one to two years for the villi to fully recover from villous atrophy, and the older the patient, the slower the recovery. However, if you haven't noticed much improvement in your health within two to three months, or if eliminating gluten has only partially resolved your symptoms, you may have other problems as well. See Chapter 12 for more information on this subject.

Current and Future Treatments

As we've clearly stated, there is no shortcut to dealing with gluten intolerance. The treatment is already known: eliminating gluten from you diet. However, this has not stopped people from trying to develop products to treat gluten intolerance.

There are drugs in the pipeline that are being talked about as potential treatments for celiac disease. These drugs will not cure celiac disease, and it is unlikely that they will be able to completely block all of the consequences of this condition. They will only help to decrease some of the damage that celiac disease causes. It's easy to get caught up in the hype for these drugs, and they are sure to be money makers, as most drugs are. But we already know the perfect and complete treatment for celiac disease: Don't ingest gluten. Anything else will be less than that.

Zonulin

Zonulin is a factor involved in the damage found in celiac disease. Zonulin increases the permeability of the intestine and its release is triggered by gluten. Currently under research is a drug that would block zonulin's ability to increase intestinal permeability, a result of villous atrophy. It is founded on the principle that celiac disease is only villous atrophy. By definition this is true, but as we discussed earlier in this book, gluten intolerance is a far broader issue. It is unlikely that such a drug will be as effective as avoiding gluten in preventing villous atrophy and it may have no effect on many of the other symptoms of gluten intolerance. It would simply be a patch for a symptom of gluten intolerance. It will not cure celiac disease. Its effectiveness will be entirely dependent upon taking it indefinitely if you choose to continue to ingest gluten. It is also highly probable that, like almost all drugs, it will have potential side effects. The one positive note about this drug is that, in conjunction with a gluten-free diet, it might improve the outcome of healing villous atrophy in those having difficulty recovering from celiac disease.

Vaccinations

Researchers are also trying to develop a vaccination for celiac disease. Vaccinations are traditionally used for viruses such as the flu, hepatitis, measles, and so on. They introduce a substance to your body so that your immune system can identify it and prepare for it. Later, if you are exposed to that substance, your body will be better able to eliminate it and therefore you won't be harmed.

Vaccinations for viruses make sense. But creating a vaccination for a food allergy is a much different issue. Your immune system can't wipe out a food if you keep reintroducing it into your body. All it can do is create a hyperactive immune response that will never end as long as you keep reintroducing the problem. That is not a cure.

Now let's say that the vaccination is meant to prevent the immune system from attacking the villi of your small intestine, an autoimmune problem. Maybe the vaccine generates a response against other antibodies that your body is producing, such as the tissue transglutaminase antibody. You still have the same problem. As long as you keep eating gluten, you have to keep blocking the response to it. It's not a cure; it's an attempt to treat a symptom. And it doesn't prevent the many other problems associated with gluten intolerance that are not related to villous atrophy.

Digestive Enzymes

Some enzyme products are designed specifically to aid in the digestion of gluten. One of these, Glutenzyme (available at www. IBSTreatmentCenter.com or www.glutenzyme.com; both lead to the same place), may be especially helpful when you accidentally ingest gluten. If taken early enough, it can help your body digest the gluten and potentially reduce its negative effects. It is not intended to be a substitute for the avoidance of gluten, nor is it a cure for gluten intolerance.

Summary

Treating a gluten intolerance or a wheat allergy is both very simple and very complex. It is simple in that one must merely avoid a particular food component or grain in order to feel better and to heal. But it is complex because that food component or grain is used in hundreds of different ways and in hundreds of different products. It is also complicated by human emotion and habits, two factors that play a very strong role in determining our diet and, for some people, provide the greatest challenge in avoiding these grains. Yet thousands of people successfully enjoy a gluten-free lifestyle and find it well worth the effort. Many even find it enjoyable, making a game out of it. Hopefully you'll get some satisfaction out of knowing that you can control your health.

But what if you are excellent at avoiding gluten yet still do not notice major or consistent improvements in your health? This is common and there are many logical reasons for it. Chapter 12 will cover this issue in great detail. But first, in Chapter 10, we'll address some of the more common problems found in people who have a gluten intolerance.

Problems Common in Gluten Intolerance: Anemia, Iron Deficiency, Hypothyroidism, and Osteoporosis

Make the most of yourself,
for that is all there is of you.

—Ralph Waldo Emerson (1803–1882),
philosopher and writer

We discussed in Chapter 3 that gluten intolerance can cause malabsorption. If your immune system is attacking your food, as it is if you are gluten intolerant, then you are likely not digesting that food properly, nor are you absorbing its nutrients as you normally would. This can be the case even if you don't have noticeable digestive problems. Malabsorption is especially common with celiac disease because of the damage that is done to the villi of the small intestine, where many vitamins and minerals are absorbed. But malabsorption is also found in other forms of gluten intolerance.

Malabsorption can lead to a number of vitamin and/or mineral deficiencies, which in turn lead to other problems. Avoiding gluten and letting your digestive tract heal is the first and most important step to improving your nutritional status. The second step is eating a healthy diet full of vegetables, good proteins, and good fats, which will be discussed more in the next chapter. In this chapter, we will discuss some specific nutritional deficiencies commonly associated with gluten intolerance, as well as hypothyroidism, which, while not necessarily due to a nutritional deficiency, is also commonly associated with gluten intolerance.

Iron Deficiency, Anemia, and Fatigue

Anemia is a disorder in which there is a problem with the formation of red blood cells. Your body starts making fewer red blood cells and/or the ones it makes are poorly formed. Anemia is fairly common in the general population and is even more common in gluten intolerant people. It is evaluated by running a simple blood test called a complete blood count (CBC).

Anemia causes fatigue. Because your red blood cells are responsible for carrying oxygen throughout your body, if there are not enough of them or if they are not properly formed, they carry less oxygen to your cells than they normally would. Less oxygen, of course, results in fatigue and poor cognitive function.

There are many different types of anemia, the most common being *iron deficiency*, *vitamin B12 deficiency*, and *folic acid deficiency anemias*. Let's take a closer look at each of these.

Iron Deficiency Anemia

Iron deficiency anemia shows up on your CBC as a low red blood cell (RBC) count, a low hematocrit (Hct), or a low hemoglobin (Hgb). However, low iron status can be diagnosed long before it becomes anemia by measuring your level of *ferritin*, an iron-containing protein complex. Iron is stored in your tissues, particularly in the liver, spleen, and bone marrow, in the form of ferritin.

Ferritin decreases long before iron deficiency anemia shows up on your CBC. Therefore, measuring ferritin is the optimal way to determine your actual iron status. While ferritin levels do not necessarily indicate whether or not you are anemic, they do give an excellent indication of whether or not you are likely to develop iron deficiency anemia in the near future.

Your ferritin level can be measured with a simple blood test. A satisfactory ferritin level is generally over 50, a ferritin level less than 30 can indicate iron deficiency, and one less than 18 can indicate *absent* iron stores, but these numbers vary depending on the lab and the reference source. If you have an elevated ferritin level, this may indicate the need for further testing in order to rule out iron overload, also known as *hemochromatosis*. You need not take iron in order to experience iron overload. Although this problem is fairly uncommon, a small percentage of people have a genetic propensity to store too much iron.

If you do not adequately raise your ferritin level, then you are much more susceptible to becoming anemic and may have difficulty breaking out of a cycle of frequent anemia. Or you may be "borderline anemic," which can also cause fatigue. Borderline anemia is still anemia, and treating it will make you feel much better.

✦ Supplementing with Iron

In most cases iron deficiency anemia responds fairly rapidly to iron supplementation. However, it can take 6 to 12 months of supplementation to increase your iron stores (ferritin) to an adequate level, depending on how iron deficient you are. Therefore, even if your CBC is normal, it is important to continue to take iron until your ferritin level is satisfactory, somewhere in the middle of the normal range.

It is important to monitor your iron supplementation with follow-up blood tests to check your CBC and your ferritin. This is necessary in order to determine that the treatment is working, that you reach an adequate ferritin level, and that you do not take too much iron.

Never take iron supplements unless blood tests demonstrate that you are deficient in iron. Excess iron can cause symptoms similar to iron deficiency and can be very toxic, leading to liver damage.

✦ Low-Quality Iron Versus High-Quality Iron

Low-quality iron supplements, such as iron oxide and iron sulfate, are poorly absorbed and often cause digestive problems such as an upset stomach and constipation. In many cases these problems can be avoided by using other forms of iron. Liquid iron and time-released iron capsules (such as Slow FE, commonly available at drug stores) are less likely to cause digestive upset. High-quality iron generally comes in the form of iron picolinate, iron glycinate, or iron citrate, which are much better absorbed and tend not to cause as many side effects. If you are having trouble finding a satisfactory iron product, you can try Ferrasorb by Thorne or Liquid Iron by NF Formulas, available at www.IBSTreatmentCenter.com.

It is wise to include folic acid and vitamin B12 in your iron supplement because these nutrients are also required to form red blood cells. It is also recommended that you take 500 mg of vitamin C at the same time that you take your iron supplement because vitamin C enhances the absorption of iron.

Vitamin B12 and Folic Acid Deficiency Anemias

Vitamin B12 and folic acid deficiency anemias both involve enlarged red blood cells. They look essentially the same on the CBC, with an elevated mean corpuscular volume (MCV) and sometimes elevated mean corpuscular hemoglobin (MCH) measurements. Therefore, it can be difficult to know which deficiency a person has. It is possible to measure levels of vitamin B12 and folic acid, but if there is any doubt about whether or not it is a vitamin B12 or folic acid deficiency, it may be easier to simply take both at the same time.

The gluten-free diet can be lower in B vitamins, which include folic acid, B12, and several other B vitamins. Gluten-free grains are not necessarily supplemented with B vitamins in the same way that gluten-containing cereal grain products are, such as breads.

But you will get your B vitamins if you eat a lot of vegetables, which are also good for you for numerous other reasons. However, this may be one reason to take a high-quality multivitamin and mineral supplement, which will be discussed in the next chapter.

Vitamin B12 and folic acid can both be taken orally (by mouth). However, deficiencies in vitamin B12 can be difficult to correct with oral supplements because vitamin B12 is not absorbed well in the digestive tract; thus, high doses may be needed over a long period of time in order to increase B12 levels satisfactorily. B12 injections are much more effective for correcting B12 levels and increasing the amount of B12 stored in your body.

Folic acid should be taken orally in a dose of about 400 micrograms (mcg) twice a day. Vitamin B12 can be taken at about 1000 mcg per day. Your doctor will usually prescribe these for you and determine how long you should take them, and will provide you with B12 injections if necessary.

If you have any one of these types of anemia, taking steps to correct it will usually help you start to feel better within days. Even so, be sure to continue taking the required supplements for their entire course. Because anemia is so common, can be so easily discovered and treated, and has such a profound effect on a person's well-being, people with newly diagnosed gluten intolerance should always be tested for it.

Osteoporosis

Osteoporosis is low bone density. Anyone diagnosed with celiac disease at the age of 20 or older should have his or her bone density checked, because it has been found that the malabsorption caused by celiac disease can lead to osteoporosis. Whether or not other forms of gluten intolerance have the same effect has not yet been investigated, so is not clear whether or not people with non-celiac forms of gluten intolerance should have their bone density checked at an early age.

There are several different ways to check bone density, such as with heel and wrist tests, but these are inferior to the DEXA scan and specialized CT scans, which typically measures bone density at the hip and the lower back. These are the only true tests of bone density.

Prevalence

In the United States, approximately 10 million people have osteoporosis and another 18 million have been found to have low bone mass (*osteopenia*), the precursor to osteoporosis. One third to one half of all postmenopausal women will develop osteoporosis. One third of all women over 50 will suffer a fracture due to osteoporosis. Approximately 1.5 million fractures occur annually due to osteoporosis, leading to about 50,000 deaths.

Causes and Risk Factors

Osteoporosis has several potential causes:

+ Malabsorption due to food allergies, especially celiac disease

+ Cigarette smoking (increases bone loss)

+ Long-term use of steroid and corticosteroid medications, which decrease calcium absorption and bone building

+ Menopause, which leads to approximately 3% bone loss per year for ten years

+ Lack of weight bearing exercise

+ Family history of osteoporosis

+ Caffeine, which in quantities greater than 18 ounces per day accelerates bone loss

+ Excessive alcohol intake

+ Vitamin and mineral deficiencies

+ Hyperthyroidism and hyperparathyroidism

Notice that the lack of milk or dairy products in your diet does not contribute to low bone density. This is a myth perpetuated by the dairy industry. Most animals have very strong bones and they do not ingest dairy products throughout their lives. And people who live in countries where dairy is not a common part of the diet do not experience an increased risk of low bone density.

Prevention

The following steps contribute to strong bones and will help prevent the development of low bone density:

+ Eat lots of dark leafy green vegetables, which are high in numerous vitamins and minerals, including calcium. Sardines, salmon, and soybeans are also high in calcium.

+ Take in plenty of vitamin D. Good sources include cod liver oil, fish, eggs, animal fat, and sun exposure in summer.

+ Get regular weight-bearing exercise. Walking 30 minutes a day is the minimum recommendation, but weight lifting is the optimal exercise and is necessary to maintain upper-body bone density.

+ To prevent postmenopausal osteoporosis, take adequate calcium, magnesium, vitamin D and other important minerals discussed below and do regular weight-bearing exercise *prior to* and after menopause.

Milk and dairy products are not a good source of absorbable calcium or vitamin D. You should not increase them in your diet nor rely upon them for improving bone density.

Treatment

One of the biggest myths in medicine is that improving bone density can be accomplished simply by taking calcium. Bone density is about much more than just calcium. For example, we are now becoming aware of the importance of vitamin D to bone health. There are also medications available to help when dietary changes alone are not enough to adequately build bone density.

✦ Vitamins and Minerals

Several vitamins and minerals are involved in the health of your bones. The following vitamins and minerals are recommended; the dosages stated are for an average-sized adult. However, you should confirm these requirements with your physician or nutritionist, as individual needs vary.

- ✦ Vitamin D3 (cholecalciferol): 1000 IUs per day in October through April for those living in the northern half of the United States

- ✦ Calcium (citrate, malate, aspartate, or gluconate, but not calcium carbonate, which is poorly absorbed): 300–400 milligrams (mg) twice per day

- ✦ Magnesium (citrate): 500 mg per day

- ✦ Zinc: 15–30 mg per day

- ✦ Selenium: 200 mcg per day

✦ Boron: 2–4 mg per day

✦ Vitamin K: 100 mcg per day

✦ Manganese: 1 mg per day

✦ Vitamin C: 100 mg per day

✦ Silica (often from the plant equisetum): 50 mg equisetum per day

Many of these vitamins and minerals will be found in a high-quality multivitamin (see the next chapter). Oscap, a very high-quality and hypoallergenic bone density product, is specifically designed to combine with a high-quality multivitamin and is available at www.IBSTreatmentCenter.com.

✦ The Importance of Vitamin D

Vitamin D, which is required for the absorption of calcium from the gut, is made in the skin as a result of sun exposure. People with a low vitamin D level have a significantly reduced ability to absorb calcium. Recent research shows that almost everyone living north of the 40th parallel (that is, the northern half of the United States) is deficient in vitamin D during the winter due to a lack of sun exposure. To give you an idea of how much vitamin D must be taken to make up for this lack of sunshine, it has been shown that the average person spending a fair amount of time outside in the summer produces approximately 2,800 IUs of vitamin D per day.

Further research has demonstrated that synthetic vitamin D2, which is added to milk, is not adequate to make up for this. Vitamin D2 must be converted by the body into vitamin D3, which is the active form of vitamin D that your body makes on its own. Prescription vitamin D2 products such as Drisdol and Calciferol are also synthetic versions of vitamin D2 and are often prescribed

155

in very high doses of 50,000 units per week. Because vitamin D2 is not easily converted into vitamin D3, it is vastly inferior to natural vitamin D3 (cholecalciferol), which is a widely available supplement and does not require a prescription. (Vitamin D is available at www.IBSTreatmentCenter.com.)

Vitamin D can be measured in the blood and should be tested as 25(OH) vitamin D. The established normal range for vitamin D used by most labs is 10 to 65 nanograms/milliliter (ng/ml). However, recent studies show that those with a vitamin D level of 30 ng/ml absorb 65% more calcium than those with a vitamin D level of 20 ng/ml. Therefore, a desirable level of at least 40 ng/ml has been proposed, and the optimal level may be closer to 100 ng/ml.

✦ Medications

This book does not advocate medication, but it can be very difficult to significantly increase bone density once it has progressed to osteoporosis. If you have osteoporosis, you should discuss pharmaceutical options with your doctor in addition to improving your diet, increasing your amount of exercise, and taking supplements.

The following are some of the most commonly available bone loss drugs:

- ✦ Fosamax (alendronate) — This drug inhibits bone loss and reduces fracture rates by about 50%. It must be taken on empty stomach and has several potential side effects, some very severe. These should be discussed with your doctor.

- ✦ Actonel (risedronate) — This drug is similar to Fosamax in its effectiveness at restoring bone density. It also has a variety of potential side effects.

✦ Evista (raloxifene) — This selective estrogen receptor modulator decreases fracture risk by 40 to 50%. However, it increases the risk of deep vein thrombosis, a potentially life-threatening condition. Side effects include heartburn and stomach pain.

Hypothyroidism

The *thyroid gland* sits in front of your throat, just above where your clavicles meet your sternum. Where it is located isn't nearly as important as what it does. Your thyroid gland essentially regulates your metabolic rate. By producing thyroid hormones (called T4 and T3), it sets the speed at which you operate, which also affects your temperature. Thyroid hormones are critical to health, contributing to metabolic rate, energy, and cognitive function. If your thyroid produces too much hormone, you will become temporarily hyperactive and then essentially burn out. Too little, and you get tired.

Hypothyroidism is usually not due to a nutritional deficiency, although iodine and tyrosine are the primary nutritional factors involved in thyroid function. It is a condition in which the thyroid gland does not produce adequate levels of T4 and T3. There are several different types of hypothyroidism, but in most cases, people who have a hypothyroid condition will feel tired, lack focus, and may experience dry skin, cold extremities, constipation, or weight gain. However, other medical conditions can be present at the same time and may mask many of these symptoms. For example, few doctors would suspect hypothyroidism in someone who is gluten intolerant and has diarrhea.

Many hypothyroid conditions are caused by an autoimmune condition called Hashimoto's thyroiditis, in which the immune system attacks the thyroid gland. This condition can be diagnosed by using a blood test to look for the two major antibodies that target the thyroid gland, thyroid peroxidase antibody and thyroglobulin antibody. The presence of these antibodies can indicate Hashimoto's thyroiditis.

Hypothyroidism is commonly seen in people who are gluten intolerant. People who suffer from fatigue, constipation, or unusual weight gain should always have their thyroid checked. Hypothyroidism is readily treatable, but there are several factors to consider when evaluating thyroid function.

Thyroid Stimulating Hormone

Most physicians measure thyroid function by testing levels of thyroid stimulating hormone (TSH), which is produced by the pituitary gland and stimulates the thyroid gland to produce thyroid hormones. TSH levels generally increase automatically to compensate for low thyroid hormone production. Thus, abnormally high TSH levels indicate a hypothyroid condition.

Unfortunately, most physicians use an outdated wide reference range when determining normal TSH levels. A normal TSH level is usually between 0.3 and 2.5, as determined by the American Association of Clinical Endocrinologists. However, most physicians and labs use a range somewhere in the neighborhood of 0.30 to 5.00. Therefore, if your TSH level increases to 3.50, your physician may tell you that your thyroid level is normal when in fact you may be hypothyroid.

Treating Hypothyroidism

The most common treatment for hypothyroidism is to take the thyroid hormone T4, also known as levothyroxine, which is sold under the brand names Synthroid and Levoxyl. The body then converts T4 into T3, also known as liothyronine, the active thyroid

hormone. T3 itself (sold under the brand name Cytomel) is sometimes prescribed when patients do not seem to respond well to T4
and have trouble converting T4 to T3. Levothyroxine is identical
to the T4 hormone that your body makes and is generally a very
effective medication.

Armour Thyroid, another medication sometimes used to
treat hypothyroidism, is a glandular product; it is made from the
ground-up thyroid gland of a pig. It contains T4, T3, and the other
constituents of the thyroid gland. In some cases Armour Thyroid
may be a less desirable treatment for hypothyroidism for people
with immune reactions to food, especially pork. For autoimmune
hypothyroidism in particular, there may also be a concern for the
potential to develop an immune reaction to the drug, since it contains animal proteins.

Rebecca and Tony

*Rebecca and Tony belong to the same gluten intolerance
support group. While they suffer from the same underlying
condition, they experience it in very different ways. Rebecca's
symptoms initially included diarrhea, weight loss, fatigue,
and weakness. Tony's included weight gain, constipation,
and fatigue.*

*Both of them have found a great deal of relief as they've
learned more and more about how to eliminate gluten from
their diets. But both of them have also had to deal with some
ongoing effects of their conditions. Rebecca told the group, "I
thought that when I got rid of the gluten, I'd feel great. But
I'm still so tired."*

*Like Rebecca, Tony didn't become symptom free when
he switched to a gluten-free diet. He said, "I do feel better, but
I'm more than ready to call it a night long before my buddies*

are. And I just can't seem to drop this extra weight I'm carry-ing around."

Because Rebecca's fatigue didn't improve as expected on her new diet, she was tested for anemia. The years of mal-absorption that her gluten intolerance caused have left her with vitamin B12 deficiency anemia. Now that she's had vita-min B12 injections and is taking a high-quality supplement, she's seeing the kind of improvement she'd hoped for.

Tony had his thyroid checked and was diagnosed with hypothyroidism. His doctor prescribed levothyroxine and Tony's health has improved dramatically. He's lost weight and has started playing pick-up hockey with his friends again.

Summary

If you have a wheat allergy or a gluten intolerance and exhibit any symptoms of anemia or hypothyroidism, then you should be screened for those problems. This can be done with a simple blood test. If you have celiac disease, then you should have your bone density evaluated with a DEXA scan. And whether or not you have a food allergy or intolerance, you will be well served to eat a nutri-tious diet and to take a high-quality multiple-capsule multivitamin —both of these topics are covered in the next chapter. Doing these things will cover the most common nutritional deficiencies and medical conditions associated with gluten intolerance.

CHAPTER 11

Optimizing Good Health and the Healing Process

Everyone thinks of changing the world,
but no one thinks of changing himself.

— Leo Tolstoy (1828–1910), Russian novelist

A healthy diet, although it sounds repetitive to say it, really is fundamental to good health. The problem is defining what a truly healthy diet is. Most people probably think that they already know what makes up a healthy diet, but when you actually corner people, the answers vary widely. For example, most people would likely include whole wheat in a healthy diet, assuming they weren't reading this book. But, knowing what we do about gluten intolerance, we can see that defining a healthy diet is more complicated than it first appears. In this chapter we discuss the key components of a healthy diet.

The Elements of a Healthy Diet

There are some basic dietary guidelines that apply to almost everyone, including those with a gluten intolerance. These are fairly simple: eat vegetables, good proteins, and good fats. Vegetables are high in vitamins and minerals as well as many other factors vital to good health. Their importance in the human diet goes back for millions of years and should not be underestimated. You should regularly eat vegetables at two (or more) meals a day, and you should aim for a large variety of colors and forms. If all you know is broccoli and carrots, then get out there and explore the entire produce section of the grocery store.

Note that in this discussion of vegetables we did not discuss fruits too. All too often these are considered together as if they are one and the same: "fruits and vegetables." Fruits do contain many vitamins and minerals and have many other healthy qualities, but pound for pound they are not comparable to vegetables. Fruits are essentially nature's desserts. Enjoy them, but ideally in moderation. And remember that dried fruit is not the same as eating whole fruit. Dried fruit is much more highly concentrated in sugar, and often has sugar added.

Proteins and fats are also vital to good health, especially for healing damaged tissue. Every cell in the body is made up of a fatty membrane and thus requires fat. And cells also require protein for nourishment as well as to build tissue. In our culture, we generally get enough protein and fat, but the types of protein and, in particular, the fat that we eat are not always ideal. Fish, an especially good source of both, is high in protein and omega-3 fats, the type of fat that helps to reduce inflammation. Nuts and nut butters are another source of both. And of course legumes (beans) have a significant amount of protein. Beef, chicken, pork, and eggs are also high in protein, but don't have as many of the most desirable fats. Keep in mind that you could potentially be allergic or intolerant to any of these. This will be discussed in the next chapter.

Up to this point we have not yet mentioned grains. You really don't need to emphasize grains in order to have a healthy diet. The importance of even whole grains for our health is overrated. The emphasis on whole grains is the result of the fact that most people eat far too many refined carbohydrates and starches, which have little or no nutritional value but a lot of calories. Therefore the current health movement emphasizes whole grains, which are far better than refined carbohydrates and sugars. While it is certainly preferable to eat whole grains, such as brown rice, instead of highly refined grains, it is very unlikely that anyone in our culture, including those who avoid gluten, is deficient in starch or carbohydrates. There are many carbohydrate and grain options for gluten-intolerant people, including potatoes, rice, corn, and numerous gluten-free bread products.

Dairy products are noticeably absent from this discussion. Although this is a topic that could fill an entire book, in brief, dairy products are not fundamental to good health. This might be harder to believe than the fact that some people get sick when they eat gluten. But the fundamental principles are very similar. The key argument, that dairy is required for strong bones, is not grounded in anything other than excellent marketing by the dairy industry. No other animal on the planet drinks milk as an adult, nor do they drink milk from other animals. There is no scientific evidence that dairy products have anything to do with strong bones or good health. In fact, the evidence is to the contrary. Strangely enough, though, many people are not capable of digesting and applying this information. Overcoming decades of very savvy marketing is very difficult, even for healthcare providers. But consider this: How do adult cows get their very large and very strong bones when they don't drink milk?

This healthy diet overview is obviously succinct. But that in itself brings up an important point: Healthy eating is actually rather simple. What is complicated are people's taste buds, preferences, and addictions. And so are all of the processed food products on the market that prey on people and take advantage of their weaknesses. Those issues are another matter entirely. But hopefully you will find this helpful. There is no point in overcomplicating something that can be kept very simple.

The Ellis Family

When her 10-year-old daughter Amelia was diagnosed with a gluten intolerance, Janet was very worried. Amelia's doctor said that the only treatment was to eliminate all sources of gluten from Amelia's diet. But how could she provide her daughter with a healthy diet that was gluten free?

From the time her children started eating solid foods, Janet, who had studied food science in college, had always thought that the food pyramid was a good guide for a healthy diet. She had always paid particular attention to what they ate, making sure that they had their recommended number of daily servings of each food group. She had always believed that whole-grain foods were crucial to a healthy diet.

As Janet learned more about gluten intolerance and the alternatives available, she realized that Amelia could still get all the nutrients a growing child needs without eating wheat or other gluten-containing foods. She also became more knowledgeable about hidden ingredients in the products she commonly bought. As she adapted her shopping and cooking to Amelia's needs, the whole family started eating more vegetables and fewer processed foods. While all but Amelia still ate wheat products on occasion, they discovered a variety of grains that they liked just as much. The Ellis family now had a more varied and healthier diet.

A few months after Amelia's diagnosis, her class studied nutrition. When the teacher introduced the food pyramid, she told the class that it was important that they eat enough servings of grain, especially whole wheat.

Amelia raised her hand. "I can't eat wheat," she said. "It makes me sick."

*After Amelia had explained her condition, her teacher
suggested that she could use it as a topic for her science
project. So she made a poster explaining that while wheat
is part of a healthy diet for a lot of people, it's not healthy
for everyone. She kept a diary of what she ate to show that
her diet was nutritious and balanced. Her teacher also
developed an exercise on additives and how they can affect
one's diet and health.*

*The Ellis family, and Amelia's class, has learned that it is
indeed possible to have a healthy, nutritious, balanced diet
without eating gluten-containing grains.*

Dietary Supplements

High Potency Multivitamins

Nothing can replace a healthy diet, not even a fistful of supplements taken every day. But no matter how healthy your diet is, it can be difficult to recover from major vitamin and mineral deficiencies that have developed over the course of many years. Therefore, it is highly recommended that at the very minimum you take a high-quality, high-potency, and hypoallergenic multivitamin. The one-a-day products commonly sold in stores do not qualify as either high quality or high potency. Although they are convenient, they have nothing to do with your nutritional needs. They are simply supplying the demand for a shortcut to good health, even if one doesn't really exist.

In order to help you determine whether or not a vitamin or mineral product is a high-potency and high-quality one, we will discuss some of the key issues involved in making vitamins and minerals. This is a very complex topic, but there are a few characteristics that can help you evaluate the choices the next time you are shopping.

✦ Potency

It is impossible to cram into one pill an adequate dosage of more than a few vitamins or minerals. This is why all of the high-potency multivitamin and mineral products include several capsules per day. They may come together in a packet or you may be instructed to take six or eight capsules per day to achieve the appropriate dosages.

Don't be afraid of dosages that far exceed 100% of recommended daily values. These values often have little practical meaning. Just remind yourself that in our litigious society it is highly unlikely that a company would be using dangerously high levels of vitamins or minerals. Consider also that your need for a high-potency multivitamin and mineral product is greater when you have a history of malnutrition due to a food allergy or intolerance.

The primary concerns for overdosing are with vitamin A and iron. If you are pregnant or could get pregnant, then you should not take more than 10,000 IUs of vitamin A per day. And, as mentioned in Chapter 10, only people with an iron deficiency should take iron because, although it typically takes months or even years to overdose on iron, too much can cause serious health problems.

✦ Quality

The number of capsules in the supplement is not the only thing that determines whether or not a multivitamin is of high quality. What goes into the product is also vitally important. It should be hypoallergenic, contain few things other than the vitamins and minerals themselves, and contain quality forms of those vitamins and minerals.

First, a high-quality product does not contain any *allergens*, including wheat, gluten, corn, soy, sugar, dairy, or lactose. It also does not contain any food colorings, dyes, artificial flavors, preservatives, or anything else that isn't required to make the vitamin. And it should contain few, if any, fillers. Fillers help to speed up the manufacturing process, making production cheaper, but they are used at the expense of actual vitamins and minerals.

Unbeknownst to most people, vitamins and minerals come in a variety of forms, some of which are more effective than others. In lower quality products, less expensive and less desirable forms are often used. Here we will discuss three examples — calcium, magnesium, and vitamin E — that will help you to evaluate the overall quality of a product.

The most common and inexpensive form of calcium is calcium carbonate. Unfortunately, it is also one of the most poorly absorbed forms of calcium. Some supplements with calcium carbonate do contain other forms of calcium as well, but the manufacturers almost never tell you what percentage of each form they are using. It is usually safe to assume that you are getting mostly calcium carbonate. Instead, you should look for a product that contains calcium citrate, which is much better absorbed by the digestive tract.

Like calcium, magnesium comes in a variety of forms. Most products contain magnesium oxide, which is poorly absorbed. Instead look for magnesium citrate, which is absorbed much better than other forms.

Vitamin E is a nice example of a vitamin that comes in two different chemical forms. Also known as alpha tocopherol, vitamin E will usually be listed on the label as either *dl alpha tocopherol* or *d alpha tocopherol*. Because the body readily uses one form but not the other, the almost imperceptible difference on the bottle makes a major difference in how much vitamin E your body actually absorbs. Look for d alpha tocopherol — it is the form that your body can utilize. That one letter difference tells you that the company is making a conscious effort to use the better form of vitamin E.

These three examples are key indicators of whether or not care is being taken to include quality vitamins and minerals in the overall product. They will help you to determine whether or not a particular product includes the forms of vitamins and minerals that are best for your body.

When selecting a multivitamin and mineral product, look for the following:

✦ Multiple capsules (rather than one-a-day formulas)

✦ No allergens

✦ No fillers (99% of it should be the vitamins and minerals)

✦ Quality forms of calcium (citrate), magnesium (citrate), and vitamin E (d alpha tocopherol)

L-Glutamine and Fish Oil

Many products on the market claim to be good for you, and many supplements do have various healing qualities, but two very specific supplements that you can use to speed up the healing of the digestive tract have a long track record and are backed by significant research. These are L-glutamine and fish oil.

✦ **L-Glutamine**

L-glutamine is an amino acid. Amino acids are the building blocks of proteins. The cells of the small intestine use L-glutamine as their primary source of energy, or nutrition. Feeding the cells of the digestive tract extra L-glutamine can make a big difference in how quickly it heals during the first few weeks and months after you stop eating gluten.

You can get L-glutamine from high-protein foods, but in order to get the amount you need to maximize its benefits, you will have to take a supplement. L-glutamine comes in both capsule and powder form. The average adult can benefit from approximately 3 grams per day of L-glutamine, ideally with 1 gram taken three times per day.

✦ Fish Oil

Fish oil is an excellent source of omega-3 fats and is ideal for healing the digestive tract and decreasing inflammation. There are many different types of fish oil with different levels of fats, but in general you do not need to look for a specific type of fish oil—any, including cod liver oil, will do.

Fish oil is available in both liquid and soft gel forms. The key is getting a fresh and uncontaminated product, and taking it in a dose high enough to really make a difference. The packaging should state that it has been tested to make sure that it contains no detectable levels of lead, mercury, PCBs, dioxins, furans, or other heavy metals or polyaromatic hydrocarbons. The average adult should get about 6000 mg per day for a therapeutic dose of fish oil. This is the equivalent of about 1 tablespoon of fish oil per day. You may prefer to take a liquid form because six to eight large gel capsules are needed to make up this dose.

Flax oil should not be confused with fish oil. Although they have some similar properties and both contain omega-3 fatty acids, the body must go through some extra steps in order to convert flax oil into its final and useful end products. This process does not occur equally well in all people. Therefore fish oil is generally preferable to flax oil.

Summary

In our culture, the notion of a healthy diet has traditionally included several servings a day of wheat products. But as we've clearly seen, wheat and gluten can be far from healthy for many people. Fortunately, it is not difficult to be gluten free and to maintain a healthy diet. And while it may be a challenge to resist the temptations of an unhealthy diet, the benefits of eating healthy food far outweigh the effort. Eat plenty of vegetables, good proteins, and good fats. For an excellent read on this subject I highly recommend the book *In Defense of Food: An Eater's Manifesto* by Michael Pollan.

As discussed in Chapter 10, gluten intolerance is associated with nutritional deficiencies, which, if not corrected, can have serious consequences. You can address most of these nutritional deficiencies with a small number of quality supplements, especially a high-potency multivitamin. It can also be very beneficial to take L-glutamine and fish oil. If you are having trouble finding these or want to save time by buying quality supplements that have been prescreened, you can visit www.IBSTreatmentCenter.com for very high quality vitamins, minerals, L-glutamine, and fish oil. All of the products on this website have been used successfully by gluten intolerant patients for many years.

CHAPTER 12

Avoiding Gluten but Not Getting Better

Education is learning what you didn't even know you didn't know.

—Daniel J. Boorstin (1914–2004)
American educator, historian, and attorney

Some people who are diagnosed with celiac disease or gluten intolerance fail to experience the dramatic improvement in their health that they thought would come with a gluten-free diet. For some, their symptoms may improve for a few weeks or months but are not fully resolved, or perhaps they improve only slightly. When this happens, their first thought is likely to be "I must be eating something that is contaminated with gluten."

The chance of accidentally ingesting gluten is great, and you should frequently re-assess your diet for potential sources of gluten, as discussed in Chapter 9. The learning curve for a gluten-free diet is steep and people are particularly prone to accidentally ingesting gluten during the first few months. However, it can happen at any time, even to those who are experienced at avoiding gluten.

Because there are countless ways to accidentally ingest gluten, it is easy to assume that if your health isn't improving as expected, then there must be gluten sneaking into your food. But even if you are taking in a tiny bit of gluten somewhere, it may not be the primary cause of your remaining problems. It is important to investigate other possible causes.

If a gluten-free diet is not helping you, your doctor may tell you that you have *refractory sprue*. This is a diagnosis often given to celiacs whose health doesn't improve on a gluten-free diet or whose health initially improves but then begins to deteriorate again over time. It has little, if any, value, since it doesn't help you to understand the problem or the solution. If you've been given this diagnosis, make sure you aren't accidentally ingesting any gluten and read the rest of this chapter.

If you are following a gluten-free diet but aren't feeling better, you may wonder if you even have a gluten intolerance, especially after learning that testing for celiac disease and other forms of gluten intolerance is not perfect. However, it is unlikely that you were misdiagnosed, assuming that your diagnosis was based on sound testing methods. It is rare to be inaccurately diagnosed as having celiac disease or gluten intolerance. It is much more common to be misdiagnosed as *not* being gluten intolerant.

Fortunately, if you are not healing or feeling better, there are numerous possible causes that are just as or more likely to be causing your problems than accidentally ingesting gluten or being misdiagnosed. These obstacles include other food intolerances and allergies; imbalances in the microbial ecosystem of your digestive tract; vitamin, mineral, and nutrient deficiencies; and thyroid problems. Any of these can prevent you from progressing on your journey to better health.

Nutritional deficiencies and thyroid problems were discussed in Chapter 10. In this chapter we will discuss age, other food allergies and intolerances, and the ecosystem within your digestive tract.

Age

Age can significantly slow the healing process for villous atrophy. While older patients can experience major or rapid improvements in their health, research and experience have shown that the older the patient, the more likely he or she is to experience very gradual improvement in his or her symptoms. This does not mean that avoiding gluten will not help you once you reach a certain age, but it may take more time to see significant improvements.

Lactose Intolerance: Not Always What It Seems

Lactose intolerance is the most common food intolerance in America, affecting as many as 30% of adults. Many people who have a gluten intolerance also have a lactose intolerance. Although they are both called intolerances, they really have nothing in common.

Lactose is a sugar found in milk and many dairy products. People who have a lactose intolerance are deficient in or lack *lactase*, the enzyme necessary to digest lactose. If lactose is not broken down, it will pass into the large intestine, where it may cause gas, diarrhea, or other digestive symptoms. A lactose intolerance does not cause problems elsewhere in the body. Avoiding lactose or taking a digestive enzyme such as Lactaid relieves the symptoms, and someone with a lactose intolerance can still drink milk if it is lactose free.

The difference between a lactose intolerance and a gluten intolerance is that a gluten intolerance involves the immune system. In all known forms of gluten intolerance, the immune system attacks gluten. This fits the definition of an allergy, and it would therefore be much more accurate to call gluten intolerance an allergy to gluten. However, it is standard to use *gluten intolerance*, so we have continued to use that terminology in this book.

The Relationship Between Lactose Intolerance and Gluten Intolerances

It is very common for people with a gluten intolerance to also have problems with dairy. In some cases, lactose intolerance is brought about by the gluten intolerance. The enzyme for digesting lactose is produced by the cells that line the small intestine. Celiac disease, as we know, damages the lining of the small intestine. This can cause you to be deficient in this enzyme and unable to digest lactose. Once you remove gluten from your diet and the damage to the lining of the small intestine heals, your body may begin to produce the enzyme again. You may then be able to ingest milk and other dairy products that contain lactose without suffering any digestive problems.

It has traditionally been assumed that gluten-intolerant people who have problems with dairy products have a lactose intolerance. If they avoid gluten and heal up, they will again be able to eat dairy products. However, it is frequently the case that these people do *not* have a lactose intolerance, but actually have a much larger problem.

The Misconception About Lactose Intolerance

Unfortunately, a great many people who suffer problems when they ingest dairy products have an immune reaction to dairy and not an enzyme deficiency. This is a *dairy allergy*, not a lactose intolerance. The reaction they are experiencing is more similar to their reaction to gluten than it is to a lactose intolerance.

In a dairy allergy, the immune system attacks dairy products, potentially causing many of the same symptoms and health problems that a gluten intolerance can cause. Eating dairy products, even if they are lactose free or if you take a Lactaid pill, will continue to cause health problems, because an immune reaction against dairy is far more comprehensive than a lactose intolerance. Unfortunately it also does not heal up and go away. It is a problem that is completely independent of the gluten intolerance and is not caused by it. And all indications are that it is a genetic reaction, just like a gluten intolerance. There is no reintroducing dairy into the diet or outgrowing a dairy allergy.

Assuming that a problem ingesting dairy products is due to a lactose intolerance is one of the most frequent mistakes that people diagnosed with celiac disease or gluten intolerance make. Sometimes it is simply a lactose intolerance, but very often it is not. If it isn't, then you may continue to make yourself sick without realizing it. Fortunately, testing for other food allergies, which we will discuss in the next section, can clarify this issue.

Other Food Allergies and Intolerances[13]

Any physician who tests for reactions to multiple foods has seen that many people who suffer from a gluten intolerance, including celiac disease, also have an intolerance or allergy to one or more other foods. This is a significant problem. Yet for many years, thousands of people have had to figure this out without the help of their doctors. As we've discussed, doctors often don't diagnose gluten intolerance, and it's even less likely that they look for other food reactions. Of course, if they don't look for them, then they don't find them.

---

13 You may be tempted to assume that other food allergies and intolerances are the result of a leaky gut resulting from the damage created by celiac disease or gluten intolerance. However, clinical experience has shown that most people who have food allergies and intolerances in fact *do not* have celiac disease or gluten intolerance. And when patients do have celiac disease or gluten intolerance, there is no consistent pattern regarding which other foods they will be allergic to, nor is there a reaction to all foods in their diet. These allergies to other foods cannot simply be chalked up to a leaky gut. They are independent of the gluten intolerance and are each important factors in one's health.

Evidence of the fact that people often react to many different foods can be found in the food industry. Many gluten-free product companies are careful to exclude other common sources of food allergies and intolerances, such as dairy, soy, egg, corn, and so on. This is a billion-dollar industry. People are obviously buying these products; there is a demand for them because people often experience much better health when they avoid these foods.

If you suffer from any of the problems listed in Appendix D, then you should be screened for allergies to other foods. This is especially true if, after avoiding wheat or gluten, your health fails to improve as much as you thought it should, or if it has improved to some extent but not completely. It is very possible that you have another food allergy. Testing procedures, discussed in more detail later in this chapter, are essentially the same as they are for gluten intolerance. If your immune system is attacking a food, then it will generally produce antibodies against that food, which can be measured by a blood test.

Any food is a potential problem. This is a list of the 15 most common food allergies in the United States:

1. dairy (including butter, cheese, and yogurt)
2. eggs
3. bananas
4. gluten (wheat, spelt, barley, and rye)
5. cane sugar
6. peanuts
7. almonds
8. pineapple
9. garlic
10. goat's milk
11. soy
12. baker's yeast
13. brewer's yeast
14. vanilla
15. nutmeg

In fact, many of these, particularly dairy and egg, which are by far the two most common food allergens in the United States, are much more likely to cause health problems than gluten. However, some people react to supposedly innocuous foods, such as flax, asparagus, or even vanilla. Every individual is unique; you can be allergic to one or more foods or to none at all.

As with gluten, if you have an allergy to any food, you must completely avoid it. Many of them are as difficult to avoid as gluten and have numerous hidden sources. For example, dairy is an ingredient in many different foods, often in the form of whey, casein, or butter. You may not notice any improvement in your health until you thoroughly examine your diet and completely remove all of the offending foods, not just gluten.

Unfortunately, it can be difficult to find a physician and a lab that can provide you with this kind of testing and are qualified to do it. Traditional allergists are no more skilled at diagnosing most chronic food allergies than they are at determining whether or not you have a gluten intolerance or celiac disease. It is simply not part of their practice. They focus primarily on anaphylactic reactions and asthma. We will discuss this problem in more detail later in this chapter.

Eric

Eric was diagnosed with celiac disease two years ago, just before he retired. For several months, he and his wife, Emily, worked very hard at finding all the hidden sources of gluten in his diet and, as a result, he felt better.

However, as the months went on, he was disappointed in his progress. He still had digestive symptoms, including bloating, gas, and occasional diarrhea. He complained to Emily that with all the effort they were putting into his diet, he had expected to be fully recovered by now. Instead, it seemed his health was still far less than it should be.

His doctor didn't really have an answer for him. He suggested that Eric may be ingesting small amounts of gluten in other products. Eric too thought this was the cause of his continuing problems, but he was doing an extremely good job avoiding gluten and rarely ate processed foods. He couldn't figure out where else he might be getting gluten.

Not finding this information very helpful, Eric sought an opinion from a doctor who specialized in food intolerances and allergies. He learned that his age was working against him, possibly making it take longer for the damage to his villi to heal. The doctor also recommended that Eric be tested for other food reactions.

"Why not?" said Eric. "It's just a simple blood test."

These tests showed that, like many people with celiac disease, Eric was allergic to other foods. In his case, these were dairy products, eggs, and — of all things — bananas. Once again, Eric and Emily modified his diet to avoid these problem foods.

Eric's health is significantly improving now that he's eliminated all the foods to which his body reacts. In fact, he feels better than he did even before the celiac symptoms became evident. He wishes that he'd been tested earlier, wondering how much of the general malaise he'd felt for many years was due to food allergies.

Food Allergies Versus Food Intolerances

As we have mentioned, the terms *food allergy* and *food intolerance* are frequently misunderstood and misused. They cause confusion even among doctors and other members of the medical community. Although they are sometimes used interchangeably, they really refer to two different types of physiological events.

With an allergy, the body's immune system attacks something that it shouldn't. However, an intolerance, as we saw during the discussion of lactose intolerance, doesn't arise from the immune system at all. It is important that we more thoroughly define these two types reactions to food.

Allergies

Allergies are reactions that involve the immune system. The immune system is very complex and is still not very well understood. But basically, it functions like a sentinel standing guard against foreign invaders — in the case of allergies, the invaders are allergens. One weapon it uses against invaders is the production of antibodies, which cause reactions that result in the offending allergens being removed from the body, often via an inflammatory process.

Foods should not normally trigger an immune response. Unfortunately, all too often they do, and the immune system produces antibodies that target the food and circulate throughout the body, which is why an allergic reaction can show up in such a variety of symptoms just about anywhere in the body (see Chapter 3 for a complete list of symptoms). These antibodies in turn trigger inflammation, which can result in pain and tissue damage, leading to further symptoms. The immune response can also produce excess mucous or, in the case of celiac disease, an autoimmune reaction that damages the lining of the digestive tract (see Chapter 4 for more information on celiac disease.)

It is not understood why an allergy to a given substance is expressed so differently in different people. Some people get hives and swelling of the lips and tongue. Others get digestive problems, migraines, or arthritis. Each individual seems to have a unique weak point where symptoms show up first. However, more research continues to be published that demonstrates a connection between various health problems and an immune response to food.

Intolerances

Strictly speaking, food intolerance is any type of non-immune reaction to or problem with a food. The most common example is a digestive enzyme deficiency, such as lactose intolerance, in which a person cannot properly digest milk products.

Some people have an intolerance to fructose, a type of sugar molecule. A person with a fructose intolerance does not digest or tolerate this molecule well. Fructose is found in many foods, such as fruits, and is derived from foods such as corn for use as a sweetener in processed foods. It is often listed on labels as high fructose corn syrup.

Another example is when people suffer from stomach pain or heartburn after eating spicy food. Although this can be caused by an allergy, in most cases it is simply a negative reaction to these foods that appears to have nothing to do with the immune system. This type of reaction also does not appear to be an enzyme deficiency.

Other intolerances include reactions to preservatives (such as sulfites and nitrites), colorants (FD&C colors), and flavorants (such as monosodium glutamate and aspartame). There are certainly other food intolerances, many which have yet to be discovered or defined. Medically speaking, we classify these poorly understood reactions to foods or food additives as *intolerances*; they are also sometimes called *sensitivities*, another poorly defined word. There is no technical distinction between an intolerance and a sensitivity. Both are catch-all terms.

Types of Allergic Reactions

As we talked about in earlier chapters, IgE, IgG, and IgA are acronyms for different kinds of antibodies produced by the immune system in allergic reactions. *Ig* stands for immunoglobulin; *E, G,* and *A* signify particular kinds of antibodies. Each type of antibody is worth discussing in a little more detail.

IgE Reactions

When most people think of an allergy, whether or not they realize it, they are thinking about an IgE reaction, which typically occurs immediately after contact with or ingestion of the allergen. In some cases these reactions can cause serious or even fatal health problems. Potential IgE reactions include watery itchy eyes and a runny nose, swelling of the lips and tongue, hives, bloating, abdominal pain, or sudden diarrhea. However, IgE reactions can also lead to many other symptoms not traditionally recognized as being caused by food allergies.

Conventional allergy testing looks for IgE reactions only, which means that you do not get the whole picture from traditional allergy tests. The problem with this is that most food allergies, including gluten intolerance, are not IgE reactions, but rather are IgG reactions. As a result, many people who do have food allergies don't know that they do.

IgG Reactions

IgG reactions may show up hours or even days after the allergen is ingested. They are often not nearly as dramatic as the more severe IgE reactions, usually resulting in "mere" constipation, diarrhea, bloating, water retention, fatigue, eczema, and so on. However, as we have seen, when left unrecognized and untreated, even gluten intolerance can destroy quality of life and lead to chronic and debilitating disease. And in many cases they do lead to very swift, dramatic, and painful reactions, so they should not be underestimated.

IgA Reactions

No discussion about gluten intolerance would be complete without mentioning IgA reactions. The IgA antibody test, as discussed earlier in this book, is commonly used to test for reactions to gliadin and tissue transglutaminase. Elevations in the IgA antibody are certainly relevant and often helpful in diagnosing gluten intolerance. However, it is currently difficult to obtain quality IgA lab work for reactions to most other foods, so testing for this antibody has limited practical value at this time.

Skin Testing Versus Blood Testing

For several decades skin testing has been the standard way to test for allergies. The potential allergen is injected under or scratched into the skin, and any resulting inflammation (called a *wheal*) is measured. Whether or not an allergy is diagnosed depends on the size of the wheal.

This technique leaves a lot to be desired because we don't inject food into our skin when we eat, nor do we necessarily get a red bump when we have a food allergy. Equally important, this test can measure only an IgE antibody reaction. The IgG antibody is not tested for at all, despite most food allergies being related to the production of IgG antibodies. Another potential problem with skin testing is that it doesn't always correlate well with the amount of IgE in the blood. You may have high levels of the IgE antibody in your blood, indicating a food allergy, but still not get a positive skin reaction. And studies disagree on the size of the wheal that indicates a positive result. A little swelling is considered negative.

Too much swelling is considered positive and the patient is told that they have an allergy. But how much swelling is too much is open to interpretation.

Many people are incorrectly told after skin testing that they do not have an allergy to a particular food. Others seem to react to everything that is tested. Like many tests, skin testing is not perfect. It is simply a tool that can help some people. Skin testing is generally most useful for life-threatening (anaphylactic) and asthmatic types of food allergies. It is the approach often used by traditional allergists, who focus primarily on these issues.

A more accurate way to detect most chronic types of food allergies is through enzyme linked immunosorbent assay (ELISA) testing, which measures the amount of both IgE and IgG antibodies in the blood. ELISA has been used in the medical field for decades for measuring antibodies in a variety of medical conditions. However, with regard to food allergies it is not run by your average allergist or lab and is *accurately* run by only a few labs that have very strict and very high quality-control standards.

For the patient, ELISA testing involves a simple blood draw. The blood is then sent to the lab, where any antibodies against food are detected and measured. A typical food allergy panel, such as that performed at the Innate Health Group's IBS Treatment Center, measures reactions to approximately 100 of the most common foods found in the American diet, including gliadin and the gluten-containing grains wheat, spelt, rye, and barley, as well as dairy products, eggs, corn, soy, peanuts, almonds, garlic, bananas, beef, baker's yeast, coffee, and chocolate. (Allergies to many other foods can also be tested and have proven to be very enlightening. For a complete list, see Appendix F.) The test is a direct measurement of the immune system's response to food and is not affected by what the patient ate on the day of the test. In someone with no food allergies, no antibodies will be detected. However, in a very high percentage of people with gluten intolerance, this test uncovers elevated antibodies to another food or foods. When this is the case, these people typically feel much better after removing the offending food or foods from their diet.

The Ecosystem in the Digestive Tract

If you have eliminated gluten and other food allergens from your diet and are still not feeling better, the problem may be due to an imbalance in the ecosystem in your digestive system. Digestive problems, skin problems, and perhaps other conditions are significantly impacted by the organisms in your digestive tract. Imbalances in this environment can cause serious health problems. While the symptoms experienced can and often do feel like those of food allergies, including gluten intolerance, an imbalance is a very different phenomenon and can be treated. If you are avoiding gluten but are still having problems, then one of the first things you should do, in addition to testing for other food allergies, is to have this ecosystem thoroughly evaluated.

There are three key categories of microbes that affect this ecosystem. These are bacteria, yeast (including *Candida*), and parasites. Each deserves special attention. We will begin with bacteria.

The Bugs Inside of You

Given our society's view of *bacteria* as an enemy to be eliminated, you may be alarmed to learn that the average adult carries about three to four pounds of bacteria in his or her digestive tract. At any one time, you will have several hundred different species of these single-celled organisms inside of you.

Although an antibacterial movement has been prominent over the last century, we are now learning that a sterile environment

— in addition to being impossible to achieve — is not a healthy environment. Bacteria are everywhere and our intestinal bacteria are such an important part of our health that we could not survive without them. They serve several purposes which include helping our immune system to develop, breaking down our food, and creating nutrients.

Your digestive tract is actually a teeming, busy ecosystem, and as with any other ecosystem, changing or harming one species will affect the other species in it. The numbers of each type of bacteria in your digestive tract change depending on your diet, your health, and your use of supplements or drugs.

✦ Bacteria: The Good, the Bad, and the Ugly

The bacteria inside of you can be divided into three categories: the good, the bad, and the ugly. We live in harmony with our good bacteria; we provide them with a home and food and in return they do some great things for us. Good bacteria are critical to proper digestion; are associated with lower rates of asthma, eczema, and hay fever; help to produce vitamin K and many B vitamins during the digestive process; enhance motility and the proper functioning of the intestinal tract by helping to break down food so our bodies can absorb the nutrients; and help to break down other compounds like some drugs and plant materials. A healthy intestinal system has more of these friendly bacteria than unfriendly ones. Because they take up space and are skilled defenders of their territory, good bacteria can often prevent bad bacteria and yeasts from getting established and spreading.

These good bacteria are commonly known as *probiotics*. Although products that contain probiotics such as *Lactobacillus acidophilus* (the best known good bacteria) have become popular recently, there are many reasons that taking them can fail to help, even when you are deficient in good bacteria. And it should be stated that simply taking probiotics is often not adequate to treat other problems in the ecosystem of the digestive tract. Very thorough stool testing will measure the level of all good bacteria, but unfortunately most stool testing does not. This type of testing will be discussed later in this chapter.

Bad bacteria are not as deadly as the ugly bacteria, but they are perfectly capable of making you miserable. They react negatively to food, are poor fermenters of food, and can create symptoms such as gas, diarrhea, constipation, and abdominal pain. They can also crowd out the good bacteria, depriving you of all the health-giving benefits of friendly bacteria and resulting in the poor digestion of food and the poor absorption of nutrients.

Some of the bad bacteria are considered normal flora, as long as their populations are relatively small and are smaller than those of the good bacteria. They become a problem only when this balance is upset. If bad bacteria have managed to gain territory in your intestinal tract, they can certainly cause digestive problems and must be treated. Again, most stool tests do not include an evaluation for these types of bacteria, which are too numerous to list but include *Pseudomonas* and *Klebsiella*, to name two. Very thorough and specialized stool testing, which most people don't receive, does include an evaluation for all bad bacteria.

The ugly bacteria, including *Salmonella, Shigella,* and some strains of *E. coli*, are never regarded as normal flora within the body. Ugly bacteria feed on tissue or produce a toxin that destroys it, and they cause severe, often life-threatening, conditions. Just a tiny amount of the most virulent strains is enough to begin the process of infection. Luckily, the medical community is generally good at identifying and treating most of these kinds of bacterial infections, although occasionally they too are overlooked.

✦ Factors That Affect Bacterial Balance

It is one of life's ironies that the treatment that gets rid of bad and ugly bacteria — antibiotics — is also one of the primary causes of the bacterial imbalance that leads to digestive problems. If, after being on antibiotics, you don't replenish your digestive tract with good bacteria, your system is wide open to be colonized by bad bacteria and yeast, which we'll discuss in a moment.

Antibiotics are not the only threat. Friendly bacteria can also be killed or their populations reduced by alcohol, estrogen hormone drugs, cortisone and steroidal medications, and chemotherapy, as well as by stress and even by a poor diet. Regardless of the reason, when your friendly bacteria are gone the result is often a digestive problem or even other non-digestive health problems.

✦ Yeast, a.k.a. *Candida*

Yeast, which is often found in the digestive tract, is also considered normal flora at low populations. However, normal does not necessarily mean that it's good. The growth of yeast, the most common type being *Candida*, inhibits the growth of good bacteria. *Candida* takes advantage of every opportunity to flourish, so if your system has been largely wiped clean of friendly bacteria due to antibiotics (which do not kill yeast), *Candida* will likely pounce, resulting in a *yeast overgrowth*. Once yeast takes over, it can be difficult to get rid of.

Candida can cause a huge variety of symptoms, including many of the symptoms of gluten intolerance. The average *Candida* sufferer reports about twenty different symptoms, ranging from fatigue and mental fogginess to digestive problems. But the symptoms vary from person to person. Yeast thrives on sugars and refined carbohydrates. Therefore a diet high in sweets, alcohol, starches, and refined carbohydrates only serves to promote the growth of yeast.

✦ **Parasites**

Parasites, like bacteria and yeast, can also cause a variety of digestive and non-digestive problems. They vary in size from microscopic to inches long, though most are microscopic and are found in the digestive tract. They cause symptoms such as diarrhea, constipation, gas, bloating, cramps, nausea, poor digestion, fatigue, muscle aches, bleeding, rectal itching, and abdominal pain. They damage the body by absorbing nutrients or by directly damaging your digestive tract and, in some cases, other areas of your body as well. The severity of your symptoms and the amount of damage they cause varies depending on the parasite involved, the number of parasites, and the level of resistance your body has. Unfortunately, a strong population of good bacteria does little to protect you from parasites.

Because parasites are mistakenly considered to be only a Third World problem, they are often overlooked as a possible cause of digestive illnesses. However, each year many people who don't drink stream water and don't travel are infected by parasites. Parasites enter this country through the importation of foods and products from other countries, and via agricultural laborers in this country who harvest our foods. The possibility of parasites should always be considered when evaluating digestive problems. Although testing for parasites is more commonly performed than is testing for most bacteria and yeast, it still leaves a lot to be desired. Many parasites are overlooked or considered non-problematic, in spite of a tremendous amount of information to the contrary. So again, highly specialized stool testing is more thorough than the average parasite test.

Bacteria, Yeast, and Parasite Testing

An imbalance between good bacteria and bad bacteria, yeasts, or parasites is called *dysbiosis*. Dysbiosis is a major cause of *irritable bowel syndrome* (IBS), which has many symptoms in common with gluten intolerance.[14]

Problems in the ecosystem of your digestive tract can be diagnosed most accurately with a DNA stool test that measures the presence of any and all bacteria, yeast, and parasites. Such a test will demonstrate the amount of friendly bacteria, unfriendly bacteria, and yeast growing in your digestive tract, and also tests for the presence of all forms of parasites. This test is different from standard stool tests, which evaluate only some parasites, or the truly ugly bacteria that cause potentially life-threatening bloody diarrhea, but do not cover the wealth of other bacteria, yeast, and parasites whose presence or absence can lead to a variety of health problems. A partial list of the organisms that should be tested for is found in Appendix H. Please visit www.IBSTreatmentCenter.com for more information on this topic as it becomes available.

Good Guys to the Rescue

Dysbiosis can be treated with a variety of pharmaceutical and/or botanical agents. Proper testing will generally determine exactly which agent is most effective. But it is also vital to replenish your intestinal tract with good bacteria such as *Lactobacillus acidophilus* and *Bifidobacterium*. This can be done with supplements called probiotics that contain live bacteria.

Unfortunately, the probiotics on the market vary widely in quality and effectiveness. Good bacteria are difficult to keep alive, and many products have little — if any — living bacteria left in

---

14 A great deal more about this relationship can be found in my book *The Irritable Bowel Syndrome Solution*.

them by the time you bring them home. Yogurt and acidophilus milk also contain good bacteria, but it is difficult to correct a major imbalance by using them, and if you have a dairy allergy then they are not options for you. You need the right strains of viable bacteria, in a high enough dose, in order to experience the benefits of probiotics. The best sources are typically refrigerated products from reputable companies.[15]

Summary

You should be very optimistic if you are avoiding gluten and continue to have health problems that seem to defy explanation. There are numerous known causes for this and you will be well served to explore them. The role of other food allergies cannot be overstated. Although the focus of this book is clearly on gluten, it would be naïve to think that gluten is the only food capable of causing major health problems.

Treating microbial imbalances and adding the right strains of friendly bacteria can also have dramatic health benefits. The importance of the balance between bacteria, yeast, and parasites to your digestive health and overall health cannot be overemphasized. If you would like to read more about these topics, particularly as they relate to digestion, please refer to *The Irritable Bowel Syndrome Solution*.

---

15 If you are having trouble finding them they are available at www.IBSTreatmentCenter.com.

CHAPTER 13

Finding an Answer

All truths are easy to understand once they
are discovered; the point is to discover them.

— Galileo Galilei (1564–1642)

In the beginning we introduced three people who were suffering but didn't know why. They are like many people who suffer from reactions to food. The good news is that these people, like thousands of others, have discovered what it takes to feel better and to maximize their health. Their happy endings follow. Yours could be next.

Matthew

Despite the fact that Matthew tested negative for celiac disease, his symptoms worsened. The diarrhea and cramps became more frequent, to the point where he was worried to even go out for dinner, much less on a vacation.

"I avoided going out as much as I could," he says, "and when I did go anywhere, the first thing I did was find out where the bathroom was."

Matthew also experienced frequent episodes of fatigue and felt achy, as if he had the flu. But unlike the flu, these symptoms didn't go away.

While Matthew's wife, Cindy, tried to be as supportive as she could, his fatigue and fear of leaving the house started to strain their relationship. The doctor had offered Matthew medication to help with the symptoms, but Cindy urged him to keep looking for an answer to what was behind them.

Still suspecting that his symptoms were food related, Matthew kept a food diary but found it difficult to pinpoint a cause. He decided to try an elimination diet. He started with dairy products but that didn't seem to help. Next he eliminated gluten, and after several weeks he felt much better.

Matthew wanted to make sure that gluten was what he was reacting to. He consulted a doctor at the IBS Treatment Center.

"I want to get my life back to normal," Matthew told him. "I need to know just what is causing these symptoms so I can take care of it."

The doctor told him that in order to be able to measure his body's reaction to gluten, Matthew would have to start eating it again for several weeks. Matthew decided that he didn't want to do that, knowing how sick it would make him feel if he did. His doctor agreed that it wasn't necessary. He said, "You don't need a test to tell you what you already know."

While eliminating all the gluten from his diet has been a challenge, Matthew says that the effort is more than worth it. As long as he follows the diet, he's free of symptoms. He and Cindy are enjoying a more active lifestyle again and recently returned from a trip to Hawaii.

Laurie

After weeks of eating iron-rich foods and taking the iron supplements prescribed by her doctor, Laurie was still exhausted and irritable, and her iron levels showed little improvement. Her hair and skin were in terrible shape, and her doctor still had no explanation for her anemia. She was grateful that a fecal test showed no signs of internal bleeding, but she was frustrated with her doctor's suggestion that she just keep taking supplements. She was tired of feeling like an old woman before she even hit 30.

One day at work she told Jane, the school director, "I think I'm going to have to quit this job. I just don't have the energy or patience for it anymore, and nothing I do seems to help."

Jane, concerned about losing one of her best teachers, suggested she get another opinion. Laurie got a referral to an internist, who, wanting to do a more thorough check, sent her for an endoscopy. Again, Laurie had no signs of bleeding, but to her amazement, a biopsy taken during the procedure was positive for celiac disease.

"Isn't that a stomach thing?" Laurie asked the doctor. "I'm not having any digestion problems. How can I have celiac disease? And what about the anemia?"

When Laurie told Jane about the diagnosis, Jane remembered hearing from her cousin how he had been helped when he was diagnosed with celiac disease. Laurie explained that celiac disease is associated with a wide variety of conditions and can cause the malabsorption of nutrients.

All of a sudden, Laurie saw the connection between her various symptoms. "So you mean that my body isn't absorbing iron and that's causing my anemia? And I guess when I started eating more iron-fortified cereal I was actually making the situation worse instead of better because I was eating more gluten."

With the doctor's help, Laurie switched to a gluten-free diet. Several months later, her iron levels had significantly improved, she was sleeping better, and her skin and hair were healthy. And best of all, she had enough energy to play soccer and stay in the job she loves.

But she was still having headaches and gas. Her doctor had thought that these might be related to her gluten intolerance, but they hadn't improved. After further testing it turned out that she also had a dairy allergy. Symptoms she had thought were due to some accidental gluten contamination were actually due to her immune system attacking dairy products. Although this seemed like insult after injury, she discovered that many other people have the same problem. After removing dairy from her diet she is thrilled to find that her headaches and gas have completely resolved, and her energy and clarity of thought are better than they have ever been.

Jim

Despite the fact that he got plenty of exercise, Jim continued to gain weight and suffer from constipation. He found it hard to perform well at work and keep up with his kids. He became alarmed at his increasing weight, wondering what was causing it and whether it could lead to any of the weight-related problems that had been in the news so much recently.

Before he looked into it any further, Jim was sidetracked by his mother's health. While gardening one day, she fell and broke her hip.

"I couldn't believe it," she said. "I'm not even 60 yet. I thought only frail elderly ladies broke their hip."

It turned out that she had osteoporosis. Thinking there might be a connection between this and her digestion issues, her doctor tested her for celiac disease. The test was positive.

Jim's brother, David, who had become increasingly fed up with his own sensitive stomach, got tested as well. His test was positive, too. Jim, though, didn't see any point in getting tested since his digestive system seemed to be completely opposite in nature to his mother's and brother's.

David was so relieved to find a solution to his lifelong health problems that he did quite a bit of research on gluten intolerance. After reading about this condition on the IBS Treatment Center's website, he called his brother.

"Jim, you really should get tested for gluten intolerance. I just read that it can cause all kinds of symptoms, including constipation and weight gain."

Not expecting much, Jim agreed to get tested. And it turned out that he, too, was gluten intolerant, but he didn't have celiac disease. He was one of the many sufferers of gluten intolerance who have symptoms contrary to those most people expect. With the help of his mother and brother, he adopted a gluten-free diet. Within several weeks his constipation disappeared and over the next year he dropped his extra weight.

Summary

As you've seen, there are many issues to consider when it comes to discussing and diagnosing wheat allergies, celiac disease, and non-celiac gluten intolerance. The road to a proper diagnosis can be bumpy and the journey can be long.

You may get frustrated by the lack of consistency between what makes sense and the feedback that you get from your healthcare providers. And you may be struggling to get the kind of help you need to sort out your problem. Hopefully your physician will be able to help you. If not, don't give up. Have confidence in yourself and trust what your body is telling you.

The fields of gluten intolerance and health problems caused by reactions to food are still in their infancy. We are only just beginning to appreciate the significance between what we eat and how we feel. But as you have seen, the evidence regarding the importance of this issue is significant and is becoming more and more difficult to ignore. In time, as we focus more on optimizing health, it will be considered common sense to test people for reactions to foods and to recognize that we are not all the same, with the same dietary requirements. People will continue to discover that they have much more control over their health than they ever imagined, and they will be able to resolve problems that have defied medical experts for decades. Ironically, many will be healthier without wheat. For these people, the answer has been sitting right in front of them the whole time.

Frequently Asked Questions About Gluten Intolerance, Celiac Disease, and Wheat Allergies

Can I have a wheat allergy or gluten intorance?
Yes. Anyone may have these problems.

How can I tell if I have a wheat allergy or gluten intolerance?
Proper testing will usually answer the question of whether or not you have a wheat allergy or gluten intolerance. That is discussed in this book.

Can I have a wheat allergy or gluten intolerance but not have celiac disease?
Yes. It's extremely common, and that is a primary topic of this book.

Aren't celiac disease and gluten intolerance the same thing?
Celiac disease is only one type of gluten intolerance. Many people have a gluten intolerance but do not have celiac disease.

My doctor won't test me for celiac disease because I don't have the classic symptoms. What should I do?
Find someone else who will test you. There are far too many symptoms that can be caused by a gluten intolerance to rule it out without testing.

My doctor says that I don't have celiac disease but I know that I feel much better when I avoid wheat and gluten. What should I do?

Trust yourself and your own experience. If you feel better when you don't eat wheat or gluten, then don't eat it. And read this book.

Why doesn't my doctor know all this?

For decades most doctors overlooked celiac disease, and many still don't recognize the enormity of it. Most doctors are also unfamiliar with other forms of gluten intolerance, which is why these are often missed. It's difficult to find something when you aren't looking for it.

Do I need to have a biopsy?

Not necessarily. The biopsy is often redundant or unnecessary. See Chapter 4.

Can I be truly healthy if I don't eat wheat or gluten?

Of course you can. Hundreds of millions of people live quite nicely without eating wheat or gluten.

My lab results were negative, but I know that I can't eat wheat. Why not?

This sometimes happens. Science is only a tool, and testing isn't as perfect as you might think. See Chapters 4, 5, and 6.

Is it important to know that I have celiac disease if I already know that I am gluten intolerant?

The treatment is exactly the same for both: avoid all sources of gluten. So it depends on whether or not you want to know.

Isn't celiac disease more severe than other forms of gluten intolerance?

It cannot be assumed that celiac disease is more severe than other forms of gluten intolernace. Many celiacs have no symptoms what-soever and have no idea that they have a gluten intolerance. Many people who do not have celiac disease suffer from debilitating health problems that are triggered by their gluten intolerance.

Is celiac disease the end stage of gluten intolerance?

There is no evidence to demonstrate this. It is simply one type of gluten intolerance.

How accurate is the blood testing?

It is generally very good, but it depends on what you are trying to diagnose and which tests you run. See Chapters 4, 5, and 6.

Is testing accurate if I don't eat gluten?

The testing is accurate in the sense that the result is correct for your situation. But if you aren't eating gluten then you can't detect a gluten intolerance or celiac disease.

I tried eliminating wheat/gluten, but it didn't help. What should I do?

This is a common problem and there are several things to consider. See Chapter 12, Avoiding Gluten but Not Getting Better.

How long does it take to feel better after I start avoiding gluten?

This varies from person to person. For some it takes days; for others it takes months. See Chapter 9.

What else is there to eat?

You will not go hungry! Most of the foods that are good for you are left to eat, and many companies are making wheat-free and gluten-free alternatives. See Chapter 9.

Do people crave the foods that they are allergic to?

Many people have expressed that this is true for them. But many others actually already avoid their food allergen because they instinctively seem to know that it is bad for them. So it certainly isn't true for everyone.

Information Resources

Organizations

All-Inclusive Gluten-Intolerance Organizations

The Gluten Intolerance Group of North America
(www.gluten.net)
The mission of the Gluten Intolerance Group of North America, known as GIG, is to provide support to people with any type of gluten intolerance, including celiac disease, dermatitis herpetiformis, and other gluten sensitivities, so that they can live healthy lives. GIG puts out a very informative quarterly newsletter and is best known for its *Gluten-Free Certification Organization* (www.GFCO.org), which certifies gluten-free companies and products based on strict criteria and on-site inspections, and for the *Gluten-Free Restaurant Awareness Program* (www.glutenfreerestaurants.org), which has developed strict criteria for accrediting restaurants for their gluten-free awareness and service.

Innate Health Foundation
(www.InnateHealthFoundation.org)
The Innate Health Foundation is dedicated to providing resources for people with food allergies and intolerances. It maintains the only wiki-based national listing of gluten-free restaurants, products, recipes, books, and other resources, allowing readers to add and update listings as new information becomes available. This site is a comprehensive resource for information for people with multiple food allergies or intolerances.

Celiac-Specific Organizations

American Celiac Disease Alliance
(www.americanceliac.org)
The American Celiac Disease Alliance is dedicated to improving the lives of those with celiac disease through advocacy, awareness, education, and research.

Celiac Disease Foundation
(www.celiac.org)
The Celiac Disease Foundation provides support, information, and assistance to people affected by celiac disease and dermatitis herpetiformis.

Celiac Sprue Association
(www.csaceliacs.org)
The Celiac Sprue Associaton is a member-based support organization dedicated to providing research, education, and support to those with celiac disease and dermatitis herpetiformis and their families.

Raising Our Celiac Kids (R.O.C.K.)
(www.celiackids.com)
R.O.C.K is a support group for kids and their parents for living a gluten-free lifestyle.

Canadian Celiac Association
(www.celiac.ca)
The Canadian Celiac Association is "dedicated to providing services and support to persons with celiac disease and dermatitis herpetiformis through programs of awareness, advocacy, education and research."

Recommended Reading

Medical Importance of Gluten Intolerance and Celiac Disease

Celiac Disease: A Hidden Epidemic by Peter H.R. Green and Rory Jones

Dangerous Grains: Why Gluten Cereal Grains May Be Hazardous To Your Health by James Braly and Ron Hoggan

Full of It by Rodney Ford

The Gluten Syndrome by Rodney Ford

Hidden Food Allergies: The Essential Guide to Uncovering Hidden Food Allergies-and Achieving Permanent Relief by James Braly and Patrick Holford

Living with Gluten Intolerance

There are many excellent books on living with gluten intolerance. This list contains some of the more popular ones and many more can be found on the internet and in bookstores.

Cecilia's Marketplace Gluten-Free Grocery Shopping Guide by Mara Matison and Dainis Matison

Clan Thompson Celiac Pocket Guide to Over-the-Counter Gluten-Free Drugs 2008 by Lani K. Thompson

Cooking Free: 200 Flavorful Recipes for People with Food Allergies and Multiple Food Sensitivities by Carol Fenster

Gluten-Free 101: Easy, Basic Dishes Without Wheat by Carol Lee Fenster

Gluten-Free Cooking For Dummies by Danna Korn and Connie Sarros

Gluten-Free Diet: A Comprehensive Resource Guide by Shelley Case

Gluten-Free Girl: How I Found the Food That Loves Me Back . . . and How You Can Too by Shauna James Ahern

Gluten-Free Quick and Easy: From Prep to Plate Without the Fuss— 200+ Recipes for People With Food Sensitivities by Carol Fenster

Incredible Edible Gluten-Free Food for Kids: 150 Family-Tested Recipes by Sheri L. Sanderson

Kids With Celiac Disease: A Family Guide to Raising Happy, Healthy, Gluten-Free Children by Danna Korn

Let's Eat Out!: Your Passport to Living Gluten and Allergy Free and other books in this series by Kim Koeller and Robert La France

Living Gluten-Free For Dummies by Danna Korn

1000 Gluten Free Recipes by Carol Fenster

The Complete Book of Gluten-Free Cooking by Jennifer Cinquepalmi

The Essential Gluten-Free Restaurant Guide by Triumph Dining

The Gluten-Free Gourmet series by Bette Hagman

The Gluten-Free Kitchen: Over 135 Delicious Recipes for People with Gluten Intolerance or Wheat Allergy by Roben Ryberg

Wheat-Free, Worry-Free: The Art of Happy, Healthy Gluten-Free Living by Danna Korn

You Won't Believe It's Gluten-Free! 500 Delicious, Foolproof Recipes for Healthy Living by Roben Ryberg

Gluten-Free Food Companies, Products, and Restaurants

Gluten-Free Bars

It's often difficult to find an acceptable quick snack or energy pick-me-up. These are some of the bars on the market that do not list gluten in the ingredients. Some are also free of dairy, egg, soy, and nuts.

Bliss bars	Jackson Hole bar
Boomi bars	Lara bars
Bumblebar	Organic Food Bar
Enjoy Life snack bars	Oskri Organics Sesame bar
Glutino Breakfast bars	Think Thin bar

Producers and Vendors Specializing in Wheat-Free and Gluten-Free Products

Amazing Grains (www.montina.com)
Authentic Foods (www.authenticfoods.com)
Breads from Anna (www.glutenevolution.com)
Chébé Bread (www.chebe.com)
Cherrybrook Kitchen (www.cherrybrookkitchen.com)
The Cravings Place (www.thecravingsplace.com)
Dietary Specialties (www.dietspec.com)
ENER-G Foods (www.ener-g.com)
Enjoy Life Foods (www.enjoylifefoods.com)

Envirokidz (www.envirokidz.com)
Food for Life (www.foodforlife.com)
Gifts of Nature (www.giftsofnature.net)
Glutenfree.com (www.glutenfree.com)
Gluten Free Mall (www.GFmall.com)
Gluten Solutions (www.glutensolutions.com)
Gluten-free Trading Company (www.gluten-free.net)
Glutino Food Group (www.glutino.com)
Health Valley (www.healthvalley.com)
Kinnikinnick Foods (www.kinnikinnick.com)
Maplegrove Gluten Free Foods (www.maplegrovefoods. com)
Namaste Foods (www.namastefoods.com)
Nana's Cookie Company (www.healthycrowd.com)
Pamela's Products (www.pamelasproducts.com)
Panne Rizo (www.pannerizo.com)
Perky's (www.perkysnaturalfoods.com)

Pasta

Rice noodles, corn pasta, and quinoa noodles are available from several companies and in all shapes and sizes.

Ancient Harvest (www.quinoa.net)
Bionaturae (www.bionaturae.com)
DeBoles (www.deboles.com)
Mrs. Leeper's (www.mrsleepers.com)
Orgran Natural Foods (www.orgran.com)
Tinkyada Rice Pasta (www.tinkyada.com)

Chicken Nuggets

Ian's Natural Foods Chicken Nugget (www.iansnatural-foods.com)

Martha's Home Style Gluten-Free Chicken Breast Nuggets (available from www.celiac.com)

Gluten-Free Oats

Bob's Red Mill (*Note: Not all Bob's Red Mill oat products are gluten free.*)

Cream Hill Estates (www.creamhillestates.com)

Gifts of Nature (www.giftsofnature.net)

Gluten Free Oats (www.glutenfreeoats.com)

Only Oats (www.onlyoats.ca)

Gluten Free, Egg Free, and Dairy Free

For those who need to avoid gluten, dairy, and egg, these companies create many acceptable products. Most are also soy free and nut free.

Breads from Anna (www.glutenevolution.com)
The Cravings Place (www.thecravingsplace.com)
Enjoy Life Foods (www.enjoylifefoods.com)
Envirokidz (www.envirokidz.com)
Food for Life (www.foodforlife.com)
Glutino Food Group (www.glutino.com)
Health Valley (www.healthvalley.com)
Namaste Foods (www.namastefoods.com)
Nana's Cookie Company (www.healthycrowd.com)
Perky's (www.perkysnaturalfoods.com)

Restaurants

Gluten Free Restaurants Awareness Program — visit www. glutenfreerestaurants.org.

Restaurants with gluten-free and other hypoallergenic offerings — visit www.innatehealthfoundation.org and click on the IHFwiki.

Conditions Associated with Gluten Intolerance in Alphabetical Order

Refer to Chapter 3 for a list of these conditions categorized by age and by type, such as digestive problems. Foods are not the only cause of these conditions, but in a great number of cases they are the primary cause. Anyone who suffers from these should be screened for food allergies.

Abdominal pain

Acne

Acquired hypertrichosis lanuginosa

Addison's disease

Alopecia areata (hair loss)

Anemia (iron or B12 deficiency)

Angry disposition

Anxiety

Apthous ulcers

Arthritis

Asthma

Ataxia/difficulty with balance

Attention deficit hyperactivity disorder (ADHD)

Atypical mole syndrome and congenital giant naevus

Autism

Behçet's disease

Bloated abdomen

Bloating

Brain white-matter lesions

Canker sores

Cerebellar atrophy

Chronic fatigue

Colic

Colon cancer

Constipation

Cramping

Cutaneous vasculitis

Cystic fibrosis

Dark circles under eyes

Delayed start of menstruation

Dental enamel defects

Depression

Dermatitis

Dermatitis herpetiformis

Dermatomyositis

Diabetes, type 1

Diarrhea

Difficulty concentrating

Down Syndrome

Dry skin

Dyspepsia

Ear infections, chronic

Eczema

Enamel defects in teeth

Encopresis

Eosinophilic esophagitis

Eosinophilic gastroenteritis

Eosinophils, elevated

Epilepsy

Erythema elevatum diutinum

Erythema nodosum

Esophageal carcinoma

Esophagitis

Failure to thrive/poor growth

Fatigue

Fibromyalgia

Folate deficiency

Follicular keratosis

Frequent illness

Fructose intolerance

Gas

Gastroesophageal reflux disease (GERD)

Gastroparesis

Generalized acquired cutis laxa

Graves disease

Headaches

Heartburn

Hereditary angioneurotic edema

Hepatic steatosis

Hepatic T-cell lymphoma

Hepatitis, autoimmune chronic

Hives

Hyperparathyroidism, secondary

Hypoglycemia

Hypoparathyroidism, idiopathic autoimmune

Hypothyroidism

Ichthyosiform dermatoses

Idiopathic autoimmune hypoparathyroidism

Idiopathic thrombocytopenic purpurea (ITP)

Impotency

Inability to gain weight

Infertility

Insomnia/difficulty sleeping

Intestinal bleeding

Iron deficiency

Irregular menstrual cycle

Irritability

Irritable bowel syndrome (IBS)

Itchiness

Joint pain

Lactose intolerance

Linear IgA bullous dermatosis

Liver disease

Liver enzymes, elevated (ALT, ALK, ALP)

Loss of strength

Low bone density

Lupus (SLE)

Lymphoma

Melanoma

Mental fogginess

Mental ups and downs

Migraines

Multifocal axonal polyneuropathy

Multiple sclerosis

Muscle aches

Myasthenia gravis

Nausea

Necrolytic migratory erythema

Neuropathy

Non-Hodgkin's lymphoma

Occult blood in stool

Oral lichen planus

Oro-pharyngeal carcinoma

Osteomalacia

Osteopenia

Osteoporosis

Pancreatic exocrine function, impaired

Pancreatitis

Pellagra

Peripheral neuropathy (numbness or tingling of hands or feet)

Pernicious anemia

Polymyositis

Poor endurance

Poor sleep

Porphyria

Premature menopause

Primary biliary cirrhosis

Primary sclerosing cholangitis

Projectile vomiting

Psoriasis welts

Pulmonary hemosiderosis

Pyoderma gangrenosum

Rashes

Raynaud's

Redness

Reflux

Refusal to eat

Rett Syndrome

Rheumatoid arthritis

Sarcoidosis

Schizophrenia

Scleroderma

Shortness of breath

Short stature

Sinusitis, chronic

Sjogrens syndrome

Small bowel adenocarcinoma

Sore throat, chronic

Spontaneous
    abortion/miscarriage

Steatorrhea (fatty stools)

Thyroiditis

Transaminases, elevated

Urticaria

Villous atrophy

Vitamin B12 deficiency

Vitamin K deficiency

Vitiligo disease

Vomiting

Weight gain

Weight loss

Welts

Wheezing

Conditions Potentially Caused by Food Allergies

This list includes conditions that are potentially caused by an immune reaction to food and is not limited to a reaction to gluten. Some of the conditions listed in the gluten intolerance list are not relisted here in order to save space. Foods are not the only cause of these conditions, but in a great number of cases these problems are caused by food allergies. Anyone who suffers from these should be properly screened for food allergies.

Abdominal pain

Acne

Attention deficit disorder (ADD)

Attention deficit hyperactivity disorder (ADHD)

Anal itching

Anaphylaxis

Anemia, chronic

Anxiety

Arthritis

Asthma

Bad breath

Bed-wetting

Behçet's disease

Bloating

Canker sores

Chronic fatigue

Colic

Congestion

Constipation

Coughing, chronic

Dark circles under eyes

Depression

Dermatitis

Diarrhea

Dizziness

Dry skin

Ear infections

Eczema

Encopresis

Fatigue

Fibromyalgia

Flatulence

Flushing

Foggy mind

Frequent colds or illness

Gagging

Gas

Gastrointestinal bleeding

GERD

Hayfever

Headaches

Heartburn

Hives

Hoarseness

Hypoglycemia

Idiopathic thrombocytopenic purpura (ITP)

Indigestion

Insomnia

Iron deficiency anemia

Irritability

Irritable bowel syndrome (IBS)

Itchy skin

Itchy intestines

Joint pain

Juvenile rheumatoid arthritis

Meniere's disease

Mental fogginess

Migraines

Nausea

Osteopenia

Osteoporosis

Palpitations

Premenstrual syndrome

Poor growth

Poor immune function

Protein-losing enteropathy

Psoriasis

Reflux

Rheumatoid arthritis

Runny nose

Schizophrenia

Seizures

Sinusitis, chronic

Sore throat, chronic

Spitting up

Styes

Swelling of hands or feet

Urinary tract infections

Urticaria

Vaginal itching

Vitamin B_{12} deficiency

Vomiting

Weight gain

Weight loss

Foods Included in the Standard Food Allergy Panel*

Dairy
Casein
Cheddar cheese
Cottage cheese
Milk, cow
Milk, goat
Mozzarella cheese
Whey
Yogurt

Nuts
Almond
Coconut
Filbert
Peanut
Pecan
Sesame
Sunflower seed
Walnut

Grains
Amaranth
Barley
Buckwheat
Corn
Gliadin, wheat
Gluten, wheat
Oat
Rice, white
Rye
Spelt
Wheat, whole

Legumes
Green pea
Kidney bean
Lentil
Lima bean
Peanuts
Pinto bean
Soy bean
String bean

---

* This list is subject to change without notice. Please see Chapter 12 for
more information about this testing.

Meat and Fowl
Beef
Chicken
Egg white, chicken
Egg yolk, chicken
Lamb
Pork
Turkey

Seafood
American lobster
Atlantic cod
Dungeness crab
Halibut
Manila clam
Oyster
Pacific salmon
Red snapper
Sole
Western shrimp
Yellowfin tuna

Vegetables
Asparagus
Avacado
Beet
Bell pepper, green
Broccoli
Cabbage, white
Carrot
Cauliflower
Celery
Cucumber
Garlic
Green squash
Lettuce
Mushroom, common
Olive, black
Onion, white
Potato, white
Pumpkin
Radish
Spinach, green
Sweet potato
Tomato, red
Zucchini squash

Fruits

Apple
Apricot
Banana
Blueberry
Cranberry
Grape, red
Grapefruit
Lemon
Orange
Papaya
Peach
Pear
Pineapple
Plum
Raspberry
Strawberry

Miscellaneous

Baker's yeast
Brewer's yeast
Cocoa bean (chocolate)
Coffee bean
Honey
Sugar cane

APPENDIX G

Sample Results for Testing for Food Allergies and Intolerances

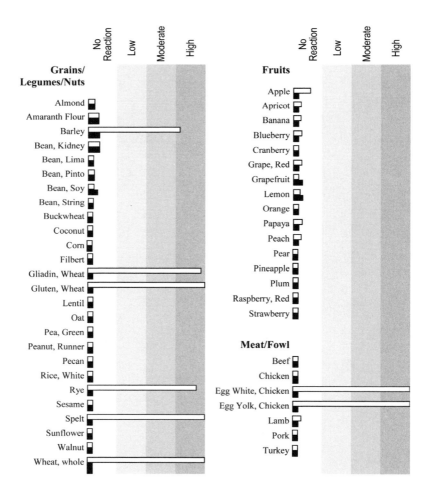

Sample Food Allergy Panel

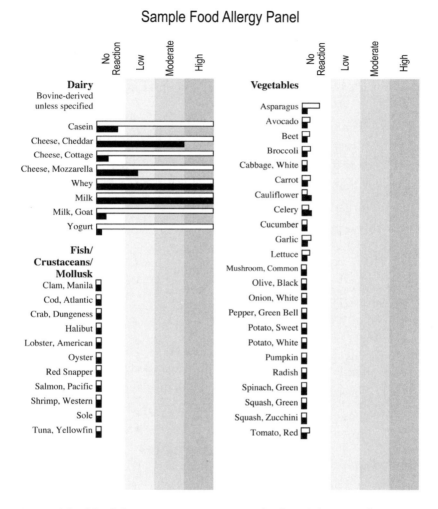

Note: The black bar represents IgE antibodies. The gray bar represents IgG antibodies. An elevation in either antibody is significant. Notice the very high immune/antibody response to all dairy products and to chicken eggs in this sample patient. Please see Chapter 12 for more information about this testing.

DNA Bacteria, Yeast, and Parasite Testing

A DNA stool assessment of the microbial environment of the digestive tract includes an evaluation of the presence or absence of the genes for all of the following bacteria, yeast, and parasites as well as many others. Most stool tests do not evaluate for many of these organisms. Please see Chapter 12 for more information about this testing.

Bacteria

Good
Bifidobacter species

E. coli (there are both good and bad strains of E. coli)

Lactobacillus species (including acidophilus)

All anaerobic bacteria

Many others

Bad
Aeromonas species

Citrobacter freundii

E. coli

Enterobacter species

H. pylori

Klebsiella species

Pseudomonas aeruginosa

Salmonella

Shigella

Vibrio

Yersinia

Many others

Yeast
Candida species

Rhodoturula species

Saccharomyces species

Parasites
Blastocystis hominis

Cryptosporidium

Dientameaba fragilis

Giardia

Hookworm

Tapeworm

Whipworm

Many others

Glossary

allergen: a substance that induces an allergic reaction.

allergy: an immune-mediated reaction to a foreign substance.

amino acid: an organic compound made up of both an amino group and a carboxylic acid group, which together form a protein.

antibody: a protein produced by the immune system to disable a foreign body, such as a virus or bacterium, or an allergen.

anaphylaxis: a severe and potentially dangerous allergic reaction characterized by rapid swelling, difficulty breathing, and a drop in blood pressure.

autoimmune disorder: a medical condition in which the body's immune system attacks some part of the body itself.

bacteria: one-celled organisms that commonly live off other organisms.

biopsy: a small piece of tissue which is removed from the patient in order to be viewed under a microscope.

celiac disease: an immune reaction to gluten that ultimately results in the immune system attacking the intestinal tract and causing villous atrophy as well as a variety of other possible symptoms.

dairy allergy: an allergic (immune) reaction to milk and milk products; not equivalent to a lactose intolerance.

dermatitis herpetiformis: a chronic skin condition characterized by itching, inflammation, blisters, and/or rash.

duodenum: the upper part of the small intestine.

dysbiosis: an imbalance of bacteria, yeasts, and/or parasites in the digestive system.

endoscopy: a procedure in which the upper part of the intestinal tract is viewed through the use of a fiber-optic cable.

enzyme: a protein that breaks down food in the digestive process.

eosinophils: a type of white blood cell and part of the immune system.

ferritin: a protein that stores iron.

folic acid deficiency anemia: a type of anemia characterized by enlarged red blood cells and caused by insufficient folic acid.

gliadin: a type of protein found in wheat and other grains.

gliadin antibody: an antibody produced in those who react to gluten.

glutamine: an amino acid found in some plant and animal proteins.

gluten: a group of proteins found in some cereal grains, especially wheat, barley, and rye.

gluten intolerance: an immune reaction to gluten.

glycoproteins: proteins containing carbohydrates.

hemochromatosis: a disorder in which excessive amounts of iron accumulate in the body.

hypothyroidism: a disorder in which the thyroid does not produce sufficient thyroid hormones.

immunoglobulin: an antibody.

inflammation: a reaction created by the immune system that is often characterized by swelling, pain, redness, mucous production, or loss of function.

iron deficiency anemia: a form of anemia characterized by low red blood cell count, low hematocrit, or low hemoglobin, caused by insufficient iron stores.

irritable bowel syndrome: a chronic but usually curable disorder involving one or more of the following: constipation, diarrhea, cramps, abdominal pain, and gas.

lactase: an enzyme used in the digestion of lactose.

lactose: a sugar compound present in milk and milk products.

lactose intolerance: the inability to digest milk and milk products due to insufficient lactase.

malabsorption: less than optimal absorption of fluids or nutrients.

non-celiac gluten intolerance: any form of gluten intolerance that does not involve villous atrophy.

opioids: chemicals that act similarly to opiates.

osteopenia: a reduction in bone density less severe than osteoporosis.

osteoporosis: a disorder in which bone density is decreased and the risk of fracture is increased.

panel: a group of medical tests run at the same time.

parasite: an organism that lives in or on another organism while providing no benefit to its host.

pathologist: a medical doctor who specializes in diagnosing disease by examining tissue samples, organs, and body fluids.

phytochemicals: chemical compounds in plant foods, especially fruits and vegetables, which have antioxidant and anti-inflammatory properties. Scientific evidence shows that phytochemicals can significantly reduce the risk of disease, especially cancer.

probiotics: bacteria that are beneficial to the body.

prolamin: a protein high in proline and found in some cereal grains, such as wheat, rye, and barley.

proline: an amino acid found in many proteins.

protein: any of a group of complex molecules made up of amino acids.

refractory sprue: a condition in which villous atrophy, or the symptoms of celiac disease, are not improved through the elimination of gluten from the diet.

steatorrhea: a decreased ability to absorb fat from food, resuting in fatty stools.

thyroid gland: a gland at the base of the throat that produces hormones to regulate metabolism, growth, and physical development.

tissue transglutaminase: an enzyme that repairs damage to the lining of the small intestine.

villi: microscopic finger-like projections on the surface of the intestinal tract that greatly increase its surface area.

villous atrophy: the wearing down or blunting of the villi, usually caused by celiac disease and resulting in a reduction of the surface area of the small intestine.

vitamin B12 deficiency anemia: a type of anemia characterized by enlarged red blood cells and caused by insufficient vitamin B12.

wheals: a small elevated swelling on the skin, also known as a welt.

wheat allergy: an allergic (immune) reaction to wheat; not equivalent to a gluten intolerance.

wheat intolerance: an intolerance to wheat that does not involve an immune response.

yeast overgrowth: an infection caused by excessive levels of yeast, most notably *Candida*.

zonulin: a protein that regulates the permeability of the intestine.

Bibliography

Many citations apply to multiple chapters. They are generally only listed in the first relevant chapter.

Chapter 1: The Whole of Wheat

Accomando, S., & Cataldo, F. (2004). The global village of celiac disease. *Digestive and Liver Disease, 36*, 492–498.

Akbari, M. R., et al. (2006). Screening of the adult population in Iran for coeliac disease: Comparison of the tissue-transglutatninase antibody and anti-endomysial antibody tests. *European Journal of Gastroenterology and Hepatology, 18*, 1181–1186.

Balzer, B. (n.d.). *Introduction to the Paleolithic diet*. Retrieved February 26, 2008, from http://www.earth360.com/diet_paleodiet_balzer.html

Bhatnagar, S., & Tandon, N. (2006). Diagnosis of celiac disease. *Indian Journal of Pediatrics, 73*, 703–709.

Brar, P., et al. (2006). Celiac disease in African-Americans. *Digestive Diseases and Sciences, 51*, 1012–1015.

Butterworth, J. R., et al. (2004). Factors relating to compliance with a gluten-free diet in patients with coeliac disease: Comparison of white Caucasian and South Asian patients. *Clinical Nutrition, 23*, 1127–1134.

Butterworth, J. R., et al. (2005). Coeliac disease in South Asians resident in Britain: Comparison with white Caucasian coeliac patients. *European Journal of Gastroenterology and Hepatology, 17*, 541–545.

Cataldo, F., et al. (2002). Consumption of wheat foodstuffs not a risk for celiac disease occurrence in Burkina Faso. *Journal of Pediatric Gastroenterology and Nutrition, 35*(2), 233–234.

Cataldo, F., et al. (2004). Epidemiological and clinical features in immigrant children with coeliac disease: An Italian multicentre study. *Digestive and Liver Disease, 36*, 722–729.

Cataldo, F., et al. (2006). Are food intolerances and allergies increasing in immigrant children coming from developing countries? *Pediatric Allergy and Immunology, 17*(5), 364–369.

Catassi, C. (2005a). The world map of celiac disease. *Acta Gastroenterologica Latinoamericana, 35*(1), 37–55.

Catassi, C. (2005b). Where is celiac disease coming from and why? *Journal of Pediatric Gastroenterology and Nutrition, 40*(3), 279–282.

Catassi, C., et al. (1999). Why is coeliac disease endemic in the people of the Sahara? *Lancet, 354,* 647–648.

Catassi, C., et al. (2001). The distribution of DQ genes in the Saharawi population provides only a partial explanation for the high celiac disease prevalence. *Tissue Antigens, 58,* 402–406.

De Freitas, I. N., et al. (2002). Celiac disease in Brazilian adults. *Journal of Clinical Gastroenterology, 34,* 430–434.

Dietrich, W. (2003, Nov. 23). Feeling lousy? Maybe it's something you ate. *Pacific Northwest.*

Dube, C., et al. (2005). The prevalence of celiac disease in average-risk and at-risk Western European populations: A systematic review. *Gastroenterology, 128*(4 Suppl. 1), S57–S67.

Eaton, S. Boyd, & Eaton, Stanley B. (1998, July/August). *Evolution, diet, and health.* Paper presented at The Origins and Evolution of Human Diet, 14th International Congress of Anthropological and Ethnological Sciences, Williamsburg, VA.

Elsurer, R., et al. (2005). Celiac disease in the Turkish population. *Digestive Diseases and Sciences, 50,* 136–142.

Fasano, A., et al. (2003). Prevalence of celiac disease in at-risk and not-at-risk groups in the United States: A large multicenter study. *Archives of Internal Medicine, 163*(3), 286–292.

Freeman, H. J. (2003). Biopsy-defined adult celiac disease in Asian-Canadians. *Canadian Journal of Gastroenterology, 17,* 433–436.

Gandolfi, L., et al. (2000). Prevalence of celiac disease among blood donors in Brazil. *American Journal of Gastroenterology, 95,* 689–692.

Gomez, J. C., et al. (2001). Prevalence of celiac disease in Argentina: Screening of an adult population in the La Plata area. *American Journal of Gastroenterology, 96*, 2700–2704.

Granot, E., et al. (1994). "Early" vs. "late" diagnosis of celiac disease in two ethnic groups living in the same geographic area. *Israel Journal of Medical Science, 30*(4), 271–275.

Greco, L. (1997). From the neolithic revolution to gluten intolerance: Benefits and problems associated with the cultivation of wheat. *Journal of Pediatric Gastroenterology and Nutrition, 24*(5), S14–S16.

Guandalini, S. (2000). Celiac disease in the new world. *Journal of Pediatric Gastroenterology and Nutrition, 31*, 362–364.

Haines, L. C., et al. (2005). Prevalence of severe fatigue in primary care. *Archives of Disease in Childhood, 90*, 367–368.

Kant, I. J., et al. (2003). An epidemiological approach to study fatigue in the working population: The Maastricht Cohort Study. *Occupational and Environmental Medicine, 60*, i32.

Lebenthal, E., & Branski, D. (2002). Celiac disease: An emerging global problem. *Journal of Pediatric Gastroenterology and Nutrition, 35*, 472–474.

Lopez-Vazquez, A., et al. (2004). MHC class I region plays a role in the development of diverse clinical forms of celiac disease in a Saharawi population. *American Journal of Gastroenterology, 99*, 662–667.

Louka, A. S., & Sollid, L. M. (2003). HLA in coeliac disease: Unraveling the complex genetics of a complex disorder. *Tissue Antigens, 61*(2), 105–117.

Mandal, A., & Maybeny, J. (2000). How common is celiac disease in South America? *American Journal of Gastroenterology, 95*, 579–580.

Mankai, A., et al. (2006). Celiac disease in Tunisia: Serological screening in healthy blood donors. *Pathologie-biologie (Paris), 54*(1), 10–13.

Melo, S. B., et al. (2006). Prevalence and demographic characteristics of celiac disease among blood donors in Ribeirao Preto, State of Sac Paulo, Brazil. *Digestive Diseases and Sciences, 51*, 1020–1025.

Milton, K. (1993, August). Diet and primate evolution. *Scientific American 269*, 86–93.

Milton, K. (1998, July/August). *Eating what comes naturally: An examination of some differences between the dietary components of humans and wild primates.* Paper presented at The Origins and Evolution of Human Diet, 14th International Congress of Anthropological and Ethnological Sciences, Williamsburg, VA.

Nelsen, D. A. (2002). Gluten-sensitive enteropathy (celiac disease): More common than you think. *American Family Physician, 66,* 2259–2266.

Nelsun, R., et al. (1973). Coeliac disease in children of Asian immigrants. *Lancet, 1,* 348–350.

Not T., et al. (1998). Celiac disease risk in the USA: High prevalence of antiendomysium antibodies in healthy blood donors. *Scandinavian Journal of Gastroenterology, 33,* 494–498.

O'Connell, J., & Hawkes, K. (1998, July/August). *Grandmothers, gathering, and the evolution of human diets.* Paper presented at The Origins and Evolution of Human Diet, 14th International Congress of Anthropological and Ethnological Sciences, Williamsburg, VA.

Ratsch, I. M., & Catassi, C. (2001). Coeliac disease: A potentially treatable health problem of Saharawi refugee children. *Bulletin of the World Health Organization, 79,* 541–545.

Remes-Troche, J. M., et al. (2006). Celiac disease could be a frequent disease in Mexico: Prevalence of tissue transglutaminase antibody in healthy blood donors. *Journal of Clinical Gastroenterology, 40,* 697–700.

Rewers, M. (2005). Epidemiology of celiac disease: What are the prevalence, incidence, and progression of celiac disease? *Gastroenterology, 128*(4 Suppl. 1), S47–S51.

Rostami, K., et al. (1999). High prevalence of celiac disease in apparently healthy blood donors suggests a high prevalence of undiagnosed celiac disease in the Dutch population. *Scandinavian Journal of Gastroenterology, 34*(3), 276–279.

Rostami, K., et al. (2004). Coeliac disease in Middle Eastern countries: A challenge for the evolutionary history of this complex disorder? *Digestive and Liver Disease, 36,* 694–697.

Saxe, J. G. (1968). The blind men and the elephant. In F. C. Sillar & R. M. Meyler (eds.), *Elephants ancient and modern. New York: Viking.*

Shahbazkhani, B., et al. (2003). High prevalence of coeliac disease in apparently healthy Iranian blood donors. *European Journal of Gastroenterology and Hepatology, 15,* 475–478.

Shamir, R., et al. (2002). The use of a single serological marker underestimates the prevalence of celiac disease in Israel: A study of blood donors. *American Journal of Gastroenterology, 99,* 2589–2594.

Sharaf, R. N., et al. (2004). The international face of coeliac disease. *Digestive and Liver Disease, 36,* 712–713.

Sood, A., et al. (2001). Increasing incidence of celiac disease in India. *American Journal of Gastroenterology, 96,* 2804–2805.

Sood, A., et al. (2006). Prevalence of celiac disease among school children in Punjab, North India. *Journal of Gastroenterology and Hepatology, 21,* 1622–1625.

Tatar, G., et al. (2004). Screening of tissue transglutaminase antibody in healthy blood donors for celiac disease screening in the Turkish population. *Digestive Diseases and Sciences, 49,* 1479–1484.

Tutin, C. E. G., & Fernandez, M. (1993). Composition of the diet of chimpanzees and comparisons with that of sympatric lowland gorillas in the Lope Reserve, Gabon. *American Journal of Primatology, 30,* 195–211.

Vancikova, Z., et al. (2002). The serologic screening for celiac disease in the general population (blood donors) and in some highrisk groups of adults (patients with autoimmune diseases, osteoporosis and infertility) in the Czech republic. *Folia Microbiologica, 47,* 753–758.

Verkasalo, M. A., et al. (2005). Undiagnosed silent coeliac disease: A risk for underachievement? *Scandinavian Journal of Gastroenterology, 40,* 1407–1412.

Vogelsang, H. (1998). The changing features of celiac disease. *Digestive Diseases, 16,* 328–329.

Yachha, S. K. (2006). Celiac disease: India on the global map. *Journal of Gastroenterology and Hepatology, 1*, 1511–1513.

Chapter 2: A Look Inside Wheat: Gluten

Abele, M., et al. (2003). Prevalence of antigliadin antibodies in ataxia patients. *Neurology, 60*, 1674–1675.

Alaedini, A., & Green, P. H. (2005). Celiac disease: Understanding a complex autoimmune disorder. *Annals of Internal Medicine, 142*(4), 289–299.

Aguirre, J. M., et al. (1997). Dental enamel defects in celiac patients. *Oral Surgery, Oral Medicine, Oral Pathology, Oral Radiology, and Endodontics, 84*, 646–650.

Arentz-Hansen, H., et al. (2004). The molecular basis for oat intolerance in patients with celiac disease. *PLoS Medicine, 1*, El.

Aslam, A., et al. (2004). Vitamin E deficiency induced neurological disease in common variable immunodeficiency: Two cases and a review of the literature of vitamin E deficiency. *Clinical Immunology, 112*, 24–29.

Aycan, Z., et al. (2004). Latent autoimmune diabetes mellitus in children (LADC) with autoimmune thyroiditis and celiac disease. *Journal of Pediatric Endocrinoogy and Metabolism, 17*, 1565–1569.

Bagnato, G. F., et al. (2000). Unusual polyarthritis as a unique clinical manifestation of coeliac disease. *Rheumatology International, 20*, 29–30.

Bardella, M. T., et al. (1999). Celiac disease during interferon treatment. *Annals of Internal Medicine, 131*, 157–158.

Bardella, M. T., et al. (2005). Gluten intolerance: Gender- and age-related differences in symptoms. *Scandinavian Journal of Gastroenterology, 40*, 15–19.

Bennett, R. A., et al. (1974). Eosinophilic gastroenteritis, gluten enteropathy, and dermatitis herpetiformis. *American Journal of Digestive Diseases, 19*,1154–1161.

Berti, I., et al. (2000). Usefulness of screening program for celiac disease in autoimmune thyroiditis. *Digestive Diseases and Sciences, 45,* 403–406.

Biagi, F., et al. (2004). A milligram of gluten a day keeps the mucosal recovery away: A case report. *Nutrition Reviews, 62,* 360–363.

Biagi, F., et al. (2006). Prevalence of coeliac disease in Italian patients affected by Addison's disease. *Scandinavian Journal of Gastroenterology, 41*(3), 302–305.

Binder, H. J. (2005). Disorders of absorption. In D. L. Kasper, E. Braunbald, A. S. Fuaci, et al. (Eds.), *Harrison's principles of internal medicine,* 16th ed. (pp. 2461–2471). New York: McGraw-Hill.

Boswinkel, J., & Mamula, P. (2003). Failure to thrive. *Pediatric Case Reviews, 3*(1), 20–29.

Bottaro, G., et al. (1999). The clinical pattern of subclinical/silent celiac disease: An analysis on 1026 consecutive cases. *American Journal of Gastroenterology, 94,* 691–696.

Brannagan, T. H., et al. (2005). Small-fiber neuropathy/neuronopathy associated with celiac disease: Skin biopsy findings. *Archives of Neurology, 62,* 1574–1578.

Buts, J. P., et al. (1990). Stimulation of secretoty IgA and secretory component of immunoglobulins in small intestine of rats treated with *Saccharomyces boulardii. Digestive Diseases and Sciences, 35,* 251–256.

Butterfield, J. H., & Murray, J. A. (2002). Eosinophilic gastroenteritis and gluten-sensitive enteropathy in the same patient. *Journal of Clinical Gastroenterology, 34,* 552–553.

Caetano, J. A., et al. (1986). Immunopharmacological effects of *Saccharomyces boulardii* in healthy human volunteers. *International Journal of Immunopharmacology, 8,* 245–259.

Cammarota, G., et al. (2000). Onset of coeliac disease during treatment with interferon for chronic hepatitis C. *Lancet, 356,* 1494–1495.

Cataldo, F., et al. (1995). Antiendomysium antibodies and coeliac disease: Solved and unsolved questions — An Italian multicentre study. *Acta Paediatrica, 84,* 1125–1131.

Cataldo, F., et al. (2000). IgG(1) antiendomysium and IgG antitissue transglutaminase (anti-tTG) antibodies in celiac patients with selective IgA deficiency. *Gut, 47*, 366–369.

Catassi, C., et al. (2002). Risk of non-Hodgkin lymphoma in celiac disease. *Journal of the American Medical Association, 287*, 1413–1419.

Catassi, C., et al. (2005). Association of celiac disease and intestinal lymphomas and other cancers. *Gastroenterology, 128*, S79–S86.

Cereda, S., et al. (2006). Celiac disease and childhood cancer. *Journal of Pediatric Hematology and Oncology, 28*(6), 346–349.

Cernibori, A., & Gobbi, G. (1995). Partial seizures, cerebral calcifications and celiac disease. *Italian Journal of Neurological Sciences, 16*, 187–191.

Chapman, R. W., et al. (1978). Increased prevalence of epilepsy in coeliac disease. *British Medical Journal, 2*, 250–251.

Chin, R. L., & Latov, N. (2005). Peripheral neuropathy and celiac disease. *Current Treatment Options in Neurology, 7*(1), 43–48.

Chin, R. L., et al. (2003). Celiac neuropathy. *Neurology, 60*, 1581–1585.

Chin, R. L., et al. (2006). Multifocal axonal polyneuropathy in celiac disease. *Neurology, 66*, 1923–1925.

Ciacci, C., et al. (1996). Celiac disease and pregnancy outcome. *American Journal of Gastroenterology, 91*, 718–722.

Ciacci, C., et al. (1998a). Depressive symptoms in adult coeliac disease. *Scandinavian Journal of Gastroenterology, 33*, 247–250.

Ciacci, C., et al. (1998b). Sexual behaviour in untreated and treated coeliac patients. *European Journal of Gastroenterology and Hepatology, 10*, 649–651.

Cicarelli, G., et al. (2003). Clinical and neurological abnormalities in adult celiac disease. *Neurological Sciences, 24*, 311–317.

Ciclitira, P. J., et al. (2001). AGA technical review on celiac sprue. *Gastroenterology, 120*, 1526–1540.

Collin, P., et al. (1991). Celiac disease, brain atrophy, and dementia. *Neurology, 41*, 372–375.

Collin, P., et al. (1994). Coeliac disease-associated disorders and survival. *Gut, 35,* 1215–1218.

Corvaglia, L., et al. (1999). Depression in adult untreated celiac subjects: Diagnosis by the pediatrician. *American Journal of Gastroenterology,* 94, 839–843.

Crenn, P., et al. (2003). Plasma citrulline: A marker of enterocyte mass in villous atrophy-associated small bowel disease. *Gastroenterology,* 124, 1210–1219.

Cronin, C. C., et al. (1998). Coeliac disease and epilepsy. *Quarterly Journal of Medicine, 91,* 303–308.

Cross, A. H., & Golumbek, P. T. (2003). Neurologic manifestations of celiac disease: Proven, or just a gut feeling? *Neurology, 60,* 1566–1568.

Dahele, A., & Ghosh, S. (2001). Vitamin B12 deficiency in untreated celiac disease. *American Journal of Gastroenterology, 96,* 745–750.

Dahlbom, I., et al. (2005). Immunoglobulin G (IgG) anti-tissue transglutaminase antibodies used as markers for IgA-deficient celiac disease patients. *Clinical and Diagnostic Laboratory Immunology, 12,* 254–258.

D'Amico, D., et al. (2005). Migraine, celiac disease, and cerebral calcifications: A new case. *Headache, 45,* 1263–1267.

Dickey W. (2002). Low serum vitamin B12 is common in coeliac disease and is not due to autoimmune gastritis. *European Journal of Gastroenterology and Hepatology, 14,* 425–427.

Dickey, W., & Kearney, N. (2006). Overweight in celiac disease: Prevalence, clinical characteristics, and effect of a gluten-free diet. *American Journal of Gastroenterology, 101,* 2356–2359.

Dickey, W., et al. (1996). Screening for coeliac disease as a possible maternal risk factor for neural tube defect. *Clinical Genetics, 49,* 107–108.

Di Sario, A., et al. (1994). Osteonecrosis of the femoral head in refractory coeliac disease. *Journal of Internal Medicine, 235,* 185–189.

Doganci, T., & Bozkurt, S. (2004). Celiac disease with various presentations. *Pediatrics International, 46,* 693–696.

Duggan, J. M., & Duggan, A. E. (2005). Systematic review: The liver in coeliac disease. *Alimentary Pharmacology and Therapeutics, 21,* 515–518.

Faizallah, R., et al. (1982). Adult celiac disease and recurrent pericarditis. *Digestive Diseases and Sciences, 27,* 728–730.

Farmakis, E., et al. (2005). Enamel defects in children with coeliac disease. *European Journal of Pediatric Dentistry, 6*(3), 129–132.

Fois, A., et al. (1994). Celiac disease and epilepsy in pediatric patients. *Child's Nervous System,* 10, 450–454.

Fotoulaki, M., et al. (1999). Clinical application of immunological markers as monitoring tests in celiac disease. *Digestive Diseases and Sciences, 44,* 2133–2138.

Freeman, H. J. (2006).Hepatobiliary and pancreatic disorders in celiac disease. *World Journal of Gastroenterology, 12,* 1503–1508.

Gabrielli, M., et al. (2003). Association between migraine and celiac disease: Results from a preliminary case-control and therapeutic study. *American Journal of Gastroenterology, 98,* 625–629.

Ghezzi, A., & Zaffaroni, M. (2001). Neurological manifestations of gastrointestinal disorders, with particular reference to the differential diagnosis of multiple sclerosis. *Neurological Sciences, 22,* S117–S122.

Ghosh, S., et al. (1998). NF-kappa B and Rel proteins: Evolutionarily conserved mediators of immune responses. *Annual Review of Immunology, 16,* 225–260.

Gobbi, G., et al. (1992). Coeliac disease, epilepsy, and cerebral calcifications. *Lancet, 340,* 439–443.

Gokhale, Y. A., et al. (2003). Celiac disease in osteoporotic Indians. *Journal of the Association of Physicians of India, 51,* 579–583.

Gottschall, E. (2004). *Breaking the vicious cycle: Intestinal health through diet.* Baltimore, MD: Kirkton Press.

Grand, R. J. (1999). Celiac disease: Then and now. *Lifeline, 15*(1), 1–2.

Greco, L., et al. (1997). Compliance to a gluten-free diet in adolescents, or "What do 300 coeliac adolescents eat every day?" *Italian Journal of Gastroenterology and Hepatology, 29,* 305–310.

Greco, L., et al. (2002). The first large population based twin study of coeliac disease. *Gut, 50,* 624–628.

Greco, L., et al. (2004). Undiagnosed coeliac disease does not appear to be associated with unfavourable outcome of pregnancy. *Gut, 53,* 149–151.

Green P. H., & Jabri, B. (2002). Celiac disease and other precursors to small-bowel malignancy. *Gastroenterology Clinics of North America, 31,* 625–639.

Green, P. H., et al. (2003). Risk of malignancy in patients with celiac disease. *American Journal of Medicine, 115*(3), 191–195.

Hadjivassiliou, M., et al. (1996). Does cryptic gluten sensitivity play a part in neurological illness? *Lancet, 347,* 369–371.

Hadjivassiliou, M., et al. (1997). Neuromuscular disorder as a presenting feature of coeliac disease. *Journal of Neurology, Neurosurgery, and Psychiatry, 63,* 770–775.

Hadjivassiliou, M., et al. (1998). Clinical, radiological, neurophysiological, and neuropathological characteristics of gluten ataxia. *Lancet, 352,* 1582–1585.

Hadjivassiliou, M., et al. (2001). Headache and CNS white matter abnormalities associated with gluten sensitivity. *Neurology, 56,* 385–388.

Hadjivassiliou, M., et al. (2002). The humoral response in the pathogenesis of gluten ataxia. *Neurology, 58,* 1221–1226.

Hadjivassiliou, M., et al. (2003). Gluten ataxia in perspective: Epidemiology, genetic susceptibility, and clinical characteristics. *Brain,* 126, 685–691.

Hadjivassiliou, M., et al. (2006). Neuropathy associated with gluten sensitivity. *Journal of Neurology, Neurosurgery, and Psychiatry, 77,* 1262–1266.

Hafstrom, I., et al. (2001). A vegan diet free of gluten improves the signs and symptoms of rheumatoid arthritis: The effects on arthritis correlate with a reduction in antibodies to food antigens. *Rheumatology (Oxford), 40,* 1175–1179.

Hallert, C., et al. (1982). Psychic disturbances in adult coeliac disease. III. Reduced central monoamine metabolism and signs of depression. *Scandinavian Journal of Gastroenterology, 17*, 25–28.

Hallert,.C., et al. (2002). Evidence of poor vitamin status in coeliac patients on a gluten-free diet for 10 years. *Alimentary Pharmacology and Therapeutics, 16*, 1333–1339.

Hancock, R., & Koren, G. (2004). Celiac disease during pregnancy. *Canadian Family Physician, 50*, 1361–1363.

Hansen, D., et al. (2006). Clinical benefit of a gluten-free diet in type 1 diabetic children with screening-detected celiac disease: A population-based screening study with 2 years' follow-up. *Diabetes Care, 29*, 2452–2456.

Hartman, C., et al. (2004). Bone quantitative ultrasound and bone mineral density in children with celiac disease. *Journal of Pediatric Gastroenterology and Nutrition, 39*, 504–510.

Haslam, N., et al. (2001). Coeliac disease, anaemia and pregnancy. *Clinical Laboratory, 47*, 467–469.

Haussmann, J., & Sekar, A. (2005). Chronic urticaria: A cutaneous manifestation of celiac disease. *Canadian Journal of Gastroenterology, 20*(4), 291–293.

Helms, S. Celiac disease and gluten-associated diseases. *Alternative Medicine Review, 10*(3), 172–192.

Hernanz, A., & Polanco, L. (1991). Plasma precursor amino acids of central nervous system monoamines in children with coeliac disease. *Gut, 32*, 1478–1481.

Hogberg, L., et al. (2004). Oats to children with newly diagnosed celiac disease: A randomised double blind study. *Gut, 53*, 649–654.

Holmes, G. K., et al. (1989). Malignancy in coeliac disease — Effect of a gluten-free diet. *Gut, 30*, 333–338.

Howard, M. R., et al. (2002). A prospective study of the prevalence of undiagnosed coeliac disease in laboratory defined iron and folate deficiency. *Journal of Clinical Pathology, 55*, 754–757.

Hwang, T. L., et al. (1987). Preservation of small bowel mucosa using glutamine-enriched parenteral nutrition. *Surgical Forum, 38*, 56.

Ihara, M., et al. (2006). Gluten sensitivity in Japanese patients with adult-onset cerebellar ataxia. *Internal Medicine, 45*(3), 135–140.

Iltanen, S., et al. (1999). Celiac disease and markers of celiac disease latency in patients with primary Sjogren's syndrome. *American Journal of Gastroenterology, 94*, 1042–1046.

Ivarsson, A., et al. (2002). Breast-feeding protects against celiac disease. *American Journal of Clinical Nutrition, 75*, 914–921.

Janatuinen, E. K., et al. (2002). No harm from five year ingestion of oats in coeliac disease. *Gut, 50*, 332–335.

Janatuinen, E. K., et al. (1995). A comparison of diets with and without oats in adults with celiac disease. *New England Journal of Medicine, 333*, 1033–1037.

Janatuinen, E. K., et al. (2002). No harm from five year ingestion of oats in coeliac disease. *Gut, 50*, 332–335.

Jelinkova, L., et al. (2004). Gliadin stimulates human monocytes to production of IL-8 and TNF-alpha through a mechanism involving NF-kappaB. *FEBS Letters, 571*, 81–85.

Kagnoff, M. F. (2005). Overview and pathogenesis of celiac disease. *Gastroenterology, 128*, S10–S18.

Kagnoff, M. F., et al. (1984). Possible role for a human adenovirus in the pathogenesis of celiac disease. *Journal of Experimental Medicine, 160*, 1544–1557.

Kalayci, A. G., et al. (2005). The prevalence of coeliac disease as detected by screening in children with iron deficiency anaemia. *Acta Paediatrica, 94*, 678–681.

Kalayciyan, A., & Kotogyan, A. (2006). Psoriasis, enteropathy and anti-gliadin antibodies. *British Journal of Dermatology, 154*, 778–779.

Kaplan, J. G., et al. (1988). Distal axonopathy associated with chronic gluten enteropathy: a treatable disorder. *Neurology, 38*, 642–645.

Karnam, U. S., et al. (2004). Prevalence of occult celiac disease in patients with iron-deficiency anemia: A prospective study. *Southern Medical Journal, 97*, 30–34.

Kaspers, S., et al. (2004). Anthropometry, metabolic control, and thyroid autoimmunity in type 1 diabetes with celiac disease: A multicenter survey. *Journal of Pediatrics, 145,* 790–795.

Kaukinen, K., et al. (1999). Celiac disease and autoimmune endocrinologic disorders. *Digestive Diseases and Sciences, 44,* 1428–1433.

Kavak, U. S., et al. (2003). Bone mineral density in children with untreated and treated celiac disease. *Journal of Pediatric Gastroenterology and Nutrition, 37,* 434–436.

Kellog, E. A. (2001). Update on evolution: Evolutionary history of the grasses. *Plant Physiology, 125,* 1198–1205.

Khandwala, H. M., et al. (2006). Celiac disease occurring in a patient with hypoparathyroidism and autoimmune thyroid disease. *Southern Medical Journal, 99*(3), 290–292.

Kieslich, M., et al. (2001). Brain white-matter lesions in celiac disease: A prospective study of 75 diet-treated patients. *Pediatrics, 108,* E21.

Kimmey, M. B., et al. (1990). Prevention of further recurrences of *Clostridium difficile* colitis with *Saccharomyces boulardii. Digestive Diseases and Sciences, 35,* 897–901.

Kjeldsen-Kragh, J. (1999). Rheumatoid arthritis treated with vegetarian diets. *American Journal of Clinical Nutrition, 70,* 594S–600S.

Kleopa, K. A., et al. (2005). Reversible inflammatory and vacuolar myopathy with vitamin E deficiency in celiac disease. *Muscle and Nerve, 31,* 260–265.

Kluge, F., et al. (1982). Follow-up of treated adult celiac disease: Clinical and morphological studies. *Hepatogastroenterology, 29,* 17–23.

Korponay-Szabo, I. R., et al. (2003). Elevation of IgG antibodies against tissue transglutaminase as a diagnostic tool for coeliac disease in selective IgA deficiency. *Gut, 52,* 1567–1571.

Krupickova, S., et al. (1999). Identification of common epitopes on gliadin, enterocytes, and calreticulin recognised by antigliadin antibodies of patients with celiac disease. *Gut, 44,* 168–173.

Kumar, P. J., et al. (1988). The teenage coeliac: Follow-up study of 102 patients. *Archives of Disease in Childhood, 63,* 916–920.

Lerner, A., Gruener, N., & Iancu, T. C. (1993). Serum carnitine concentrations in coeliac disease. *Gut, 34,* 933–935.

Levin, B. (1999). *Environmental nutrition: Understanding the link between environment, food quality, and disease.* Vashon Island, WA: Hingepin.

Li, J., et al. (1994). Glutamine prevents parenteral nutrition-induced increases in intestinal permeability. *Journal of Parenteral and Enteral Nutrition, 18,* 303–307.

Lorini, R., et al. (2003). Hashimoto's thyroiditis. *Pediatric Endocrinology Reviews, 1*(Suppl. 2), 205–211.

Ludvigsson, J. F., et al. (2006). Celiac disease and risk of subsequent type 1 diabetes: A general population cohort study of children and adolescents. *Diabetes Care, 29,* 2483–2488.

Lundin, K. E., et al. (2003). Oats induced villous atrophy in coeliac disease. *Gut, 52,* 1649–1652.

Luostarinen, L., et al. (2001). Association between coeliac disease, epilepsy and brain atrophy. *European Neurology, 46,* 187–191.

Luostarinen, L., et al. (2003). Neuromuscular and sensory disturbances in patients with well treated coeliac disease. *Journal of Neurology, Neurosurgery, and Psychiatry, 74,* 490–494.

Maggiore, G., & Caprai, S. (2006). Liver involvement in celiac disease. *Indian Journal of Pediatrics, 73,* 809–811.

Maiuri, L., et al. (2000). Interleukin 15 mediates epithelial changes in celiac disease. *Gastroenterology, 119,* 996–1006.

Maiuri, L., et al. (2001). IL-15 drives the specific migration of CD94+ and TCRgammadelta+ intraepithelial lymphocytes in organ cultures of treated celiac patients. *American Journal of Gastroenterology, 96,* 150–156.

Maiuri, L., et al. (2003). Association between innate response to gliadin and activation of pathogenic T cells in coeliac disease. *Lancet, 362,* 30–37.

Maiuri, M. C., et al. (2003a).Gliadin increases iNOS gene expression in interferongamma-stimulated RAW 264.7 cells through a mechanism involving NF-kappa B. *Naunyn-Schrniedeberg's Archives of Pharmacology, 368,* 63–71.

Maiuri, M. C., et al. (2003b). Nuclear factor kappa B is activated in small intestinal mucosa of celiac patients. *Journal of Molecular Medicine, 81,* 373–379.

Maki, M., & Collin, P. (1997). Coeliac disease. *Lancet, 349,* 1755–1759.

Manek, S., & Lew, M. F. (2003). Gait and balance dysfunction in adults. *Current Treatment Options in Neurology, 5,* 177–185.

Mant, M. J., et al. (2006). Prevalence of occult gastrointestinal bleeding in celiac disease. *Clinical Gastroenterology and Hepatology, 4,* 451–454.

Marietta, E., et al. (2004). A new model for dermatitis herpetiformis that uses HLA-DQ8 transgenic NOD mice. *Journal of Clinical Investigation, 114,* 1090–1097.

Martinelli, P., et al. (2000). Coeliac disease and unfavourable outcome of pregnancy. *Gut, 46*(3), 332–335.

Mata, S., et al. (2006). Anti-tissue transglutaminase IgA antibodies in peripheral neuropathy and motor neuronopathy. *Acta Neurological Scandinavica, 114*(1), 54–58.

Mathews, S., et al. (2000). Phylogenetic structure in the grass family (*Poaceae*): Evidence from the nuclear gene phytochrome B. *American Journal of Botany, 87,* 96–107.

Matzinger P. (2002). The danger model: A renewed sense of self. *Science, 296,* 301–305.

Mavroudi, A., et al. (2005). Successful treatment of epilepsy and celiac disease with a gluten-free diet. *Pediatric Neurology, 33*(4), 292–295.

Mearin, M. L., et al. (2006). European multi-centre study on coeliac disease and non-Hodgkin lymphoma. *European Journal of Gastroenterology and Hepatology, 18*(2), 187–194.

Melo, F. M., et al. (2005). [Association between serum markers for celiac and thyroid autoimmune diseases]. *Arquivos Brasileiros de Endocrinologia e Metabologia, 49,* 542–547.

Mention, J. J., et al. (2003). Interleukin 15: A key to disrupted intraepithelial lymphocyte homeostasis and lymphomagenesis in celiac disease. *Gastroenterology, 125,* 730–745.

Meyer, D., et al. (2001). Osteoporosis in a North American adult population with celiac disease. *American Journal of Gastroenterology, 96,* 112–119.

Midhagen, G., et al. (2004). Antibody levels in adult patients with coeliac disease during gluten-free diet: A rapid initial decrease of clinical importance. *Journal of Internal Medicine, 256,* 519–524.

Molberg, O., et al. (2003). Intestinal T-cell responses to high-molecular-weight glutenins in celiac disease. *Gastroenterology, 125,* 337–344.

Monteleone, G., et al. (2001). Interferon-alpha drives T cell-mediated immunopathology in the intestine. *European Journal of Immunology, 31,* 2247–2255.

Montgomery, A. M., et al. (1988). Low gluten diet in the treatment of adult coeliac disease: Effect on jejunal morphology and serum anti-gluten antibodies. *Gut, 29,* 1564–1568.

Murray, J. A., et al. (2004). Effect of a gluten-free diet on gastrointestinal symptoms in celiac disease. *American Journal of Clinical Nutrition, 79,* 669–673.

Myhre, A. G., et al. (2003). High frequency of coeliac disease among patients with autoimmune adrenocortical failure. *Scandinavian Journal of Gastroenterology, 38,* 511–515.

Nieuwenhuizen, W. F., et al. (2003). Is *Candida albicans* a trigger in the onset of coeliac disease? *Lancet, 361,* 2152–2154.

O'Dwyer, S. T., et al. (1989). Maintenance of small bowel mucosa with glutamine-enriched parenteral nutrition. *Journal of Parenteral and Enteral Nutrition, 13,* 579–585.

O'Leary, C., et al. (2002). Coeliac disease and autoimmune Addison's disease: A clinical pitfall. *Quarterly Journal of Medicine, 95,* 79–82.

O'Leary, C., et al. (2004). Celiac disease and the transition from childhood to adulthood: A 28-year follow-up. *American Journal of Gastroenterology, 99,* 2437–2441.

Payne, P. I. (1987). Genetics of wheat storage proteins and the effect of allelic variation on bread-making quality. *Annual Review of Plant Physiology, 38,* 141–153.

Pellecchia, M. T., et al. (2002). Possible gluten sensitivity in multiple system atrophy. *Neurology, 59,* 1114–1115.

Peretti, N., et al. (2004). The temporal relationship between the onset of type 1 diabetes and celiac disease: A study based on immunoglobulin a antitransglutaminase screening. *Pediatrics, 113,* E418–E422.

Pizzorno, J. E., & Murray, M. T. (1999). *Textbook of natural medicine.* New York: Churchill Livingstone.

Polizzi, A., et al. (2000). Recurrent peripheral neuropathy in a girl with celiac disease. *Journal of Neurology, Neurosurgery, and Psychiatry, 68,* 104–105.

Pratesi, R., et al. (1998). Serum IgA antibodies from patients with coeliac disease react strongly with human brain blood-vessel structures. *Scandinavian Journal of Gastroenterology, 33,* 817–821.

Pratesi, R., et al. (2003). Celiac disease and epilepsy: Favorable outcome in a child with difficult to control seizures. *Acta Neurological Scandinavica, 108,* 290–293.

Pynnonen, P. A., et al. (2002). Untreated celiac disease and development of mental disorders in children and adolescents. *Psychosomatics, 43,* 331–334.

Rensch, M. J., et al. (2001). The prevalence of celiac disease auto-antibodies in patients with systemic lupus erythematosus. *American Journal of Gastroenterology, 96,* 1113–1115.

Reunala, T., et al. (1987). Dermatitis herpetiformis and celiac disease associated with Addison's disease. *Archives of Dermatology, 123,* 930–932.

Roche Herrero, M. C., et al. (2001). [The prevalence of headache in a population of patients with coeliac disease.] *Revista de neurologia, 32,* 301–309.

Saadah, O. I., et al. (2004). Effect of gluten-free diet and adherence on growth and diabetic control in diabetics with celiac disease. *Archives of Disease in Childhood, 89,* 871–876.

Schalock, P. C., & Baughman, R. D. (2005). Flare of dermatitis herpetiformis associated with gluten in multivitamins. *Journal of the American Academy of Dermatology, 52*, 367.

Scotta, M. S., et al. (1997). Bone mineralization and body composition in young patients with celiac disease. *American Journal of Gastroenterology, 92*, 1331–1334.

Serratrice, J., et al. (1998). Migraine and coeliac disease. *Headache, 38*, 627–628.

Shan, L., et al. (2002). Structural basis for gluten intolerance in celiac sprue. *Science, 297*, 2275–2279.

Sharma, R., & Schumacher, U. (2001). Carbohydrate expression in the intestinal mucosa. *Advances in Anatomy, Embryology, and Cell Biology, 160*, III–IX,1–91.

Sher, K. S., & Mayberry, J. F. (1994). Female fertility, obstetric and gynaecological history in coeliac disease: A case control study. *Digestion, 55*(4), 243–246.

Sicherer, S. H. (2003). Clinical aspects of gastrointestinal food allergy in childhood. *Pediatrics, 111*,1609–1616.

Simonati, A., et al. (1998). Coeliac disease associated with peripheral neuropathy in a child: A case report. *Neuropediatrics, 29*, 155–158.

Siniscalchi, M., et al. (2005). Fatigue in adult coeliac disease. *Alimentary Pharmacology and Therapeutics, 22*(5), 489–494.

Sjoberg, K., & Carlsson, A. (2004). [Screening for celiac disease can be justified in high-risk groups.] *Lakartidningen, 101*, 3912, 3915–3916, 3918–3919. [Article in Swedish]

Slot, O., & Locht, H. (2000). Arthritis as presenting symptom in silent adult coeliac disease: Two cases and review of the literature. *Scandinavian Journal of Rheumatology, 29*, 260–263.

Smecuol, E., et al. (2005). Permeability, zonulin production, and enteropathy in dermatitis herpetiformis. *Clinical Gastroenterology and Hepatology, 3*, 335–341.

Spina, M., et al. (2001). [Headache as atypical presentation of celiac disease: Report of a clinical case.] *La pediatria medica e chirurgica, 23*, 133–135.

Staab, J. F., et al. (1999). Adhesive and mammalian transglutaminase substrate properties of *Candida albicans* Hwp1. *Science, 283,* 1535–1538.

Stazi, A. V., & Mantovani, A. (2000). A risk factor for female fertility and pregnancy: celiac disease. *Gynecological Endocrinology, 14,* 454–463.

Stazi, A. V., & Mantovani, A. (2004). [Celiac disease and its endocrine and nutritional implications on male reproduction]. *Minerva Medica, 95*(3), 243–254.

Stazi, A. V., & Trinti, B. (2005). [Reproductive aspects of celiac disease]. *Annali Italiani di Medicina Interna, 20*(3), 143–157.

Stenson, W. F., et al. (2005). Increased prevalence of celiac disease and need for routine screening among patients with osteoporosis. *Archives of Internal Medicine, 165,* 393–399.

Stevens, F. M., & McLoughlin, R. M. (2005). Is coeliac disease a potentially treatable cause of liver failure? *European Journal of Gastroenterology and Hepatology, 17,* 1015–1017.

Stockbrugger, R., et al. (1976). Auto-immune atrophic gastritis in patient with dermatitis herpetiformis. *Acta Dermata-Venereologica, 56,* 111–113.

Storsrud, S., et al. (2003). Beneficial effects of oats in the gluten-free diet of adults with special reference to nutrient status, symptoms and subjective experiences. *British Journal of Nutrition, 90,* 101–107.

Swinson, C. M., et al. (1983). Coeliac disease and malignancy. *Lancet 1*(8316): 111–115.

Szodoray, P., et al. (2004). Coeliac disease in Sjogren's syndrome: A study of 111 Hungarian patients. *Rheumatology International, 24,* 278–282.

Thompson, T. (2004). Gluten contamination of commercial oat products in the United States. *New England Journal of Medicine, 351,* 2021–2022.

Thomson, A. (2005). Celiac disease as a cause of pancreatitis. *Gastroenterology, 129,* 1137.

Tommasini, A., et al. (2004). Mass screening for coeliac disease using antihuman transglutaminase antibody assay. *Archives of Disease in Childhood, 89,* 512–515.

Toscano, V., et al. (2000). Importance of gluten in the induction of endocrine autoantibodies and organ dysfunction in adolescent celiac patients. *American Journal of Gastroenterology, 95,* 1742–1748.

Valdimarsson, T., et al. (1994). Bone mineral density in coeliac disease. *Scandinavian Journal of Gastroenterology, 29,* 457–461.

Vanderhoof, J. A. (1998). Food hypersensitivity in children. *Current Opinion in Clinical Nutrition and Metabolic Care, 1,* 419–422.

Vanderhoof, J. A., & Young, R. J. (2001). Allergic disorders of the gastrointestinal tract. *Current Opinion in Clinical Nutrition and Metabolic Care, 4,* 553–556.

Vanderhoof, J. A., et al. (2001). Allergic constipation, association with infantile milk allergy. *Clinical Pediatrics, 40,* 399–402.

Ventura, A., et al. (1999). Duration of exposure to gluten and risk for autoimmune disorders in patients with celiac disease. *Gastroenterology, 117,* 297–303.

Verslype, C. (2004). Evaluation of abnormal liver-enzyme results in asymptomatic patients. *Acta Clinica Belgica, 59,* 285–289.

Vesy, C. J., et al. (1993). Evaluation of celiac disease biopsies for adenovirus 12 DNA using a multiplex polymerase chain reaction. *Modern Pathology, 6,* 61–64.

Volta, U., et al. (2002). Clinical findings and anti-neuronal antibodies in celiac disease with neurological disorders. *Scandinavian Journal of Gastroenterology, 37,* 1276–1281.

Weinberg, J. B., et al. (1991). Extravascular fibrin formation and dissolution in synovial tissue of patients with osteoarthritis and rheumatoid arthritis. *Arthritis and Rheumatism, 34,* 996–1005.

West, J., et al. (2003). Fracture risk in people with celiac disease: A population-based cohort study. *Gastroenterology, 125,* 429–436.

West, J., et al. (2004). Malignancy and mortality in people with coeliac disease: Population-based cohort study. *BMJ, 329,* 716–719.

Yancey, K. B., & Lawley, T. J. (2005). Immunologically mediated skin diseases. In D. L. Kasper, E. Braunbald, A. S. Fuaci, et al. (Eds.), *Harrison's Principles of Internal Medicine*, 16th ed. (p. 314). New York: McGraw-Hill.

Yuce, A., et al. (2004). Serum carnitine and selenium levels in children with celiac disease. *Indian Journal of Gastroenterology, 23*, 87–88.

Zelnik, N., et al. (2004). Range of neurologic disorders in patients with celiac disease. *Pediatrics, 113*, 1672–1676.

Ziegler, A. G., et al. (2003). Early infant feeding and risk of developing type 1 diabetes-associated autoantibodies. *Journal of the American Medical Association, 290*, 1721–1728.

Chapter 3: Reacting to Wheat: The Many Faces of Gluten Intolerance and Gluten-Associated Diseases

Many of the references relevant to this chapter are listed under other chapters.

Abenavoli, L., et al. (2006). Cutaneous manifestations in celiac disease. *World Journal of Gastroenterology, 12*, 843–852.

Dohan, F. C. (1988). Genetic hypothesis of idiopathic schizophrenia: Its exorphin connection. *Schizophrenia Bulletin, 14*, 489–494.

Fanciulli, G., et al. (2005). Gluten exorphin B5 stimulates prolactin secretion through opioid receptors located outside the blood-brain barrier. *Life Sciences, 76*, 1713–1719.

Fukudome, S., & Yoshikawa, M. (1992). Opioid peptides derived from wheat gluten: Their isolation and characterization. *Federation of Biochemical Societies Letters, 296*, 107–111.

Fukudome, S., & Yoshikawa, M. (1993). Gluten exorphin C. A novel opioid peptide derived from wheat gluten. *Federation of Biochemical Societies Letters, 316*, 17–19.

Fukudome, S., et al. (1997). Release of opioid peptides, gluten exorphins by the action of pancreatic elastase. *Federation of Biochemical Societies Letters, 412*, 475–479.

Kather, H., & Simon, B. (1979, October 27). Opioid peptides and obesity. *Lancet, 2*, 905.

Kawashti, M. I., et al. (2006). Possible immunological disorders in autism: Concomitant autoimmunity and immune tolerance. *Egyptian Journal of Immunology, 13*(1), 99–104.

Millward, C., et al. (2004). Gluten- and casein-free diets for autistic spectrum disorder. *Cochrane Database of Systematic Reviews*, 2, CD003498.

Millward, C., et al. (2008). Update to Gluten- and casein-free diets for autistic spectrum disorder. *Cochrane Database of Systematic Reviews*, 2, CD003498.

Reichelt, K. L., & Skjeldal, O. (2006). IgA antibodies in Rett syndrome. *Autism, 10*, 189–197.

Schick, R., & Schusdziarra, V. (1985). Physiological, pathophysiological and pharmacological aspects of exogenous and endogenous opiates. *Clinical Physiology and Biochemistry, 3*(1), 43–60.

Shattock, P., & Whiteley, P. (2002). Biochemical aspects in autism spectrum disorders: updating the opioid-excess theory and presenting new opportunities for biomedical intervention. *Expert Opinion on Therapeutic Targets, 6*(12), 175–183.

Teschemacher, H. (2003). Opioid receptor ligands derived from food proteins. *Current Pharmaceutical Design, 9*, 1331–1344.

Yoshikawa, M., et al. (2003). Delta opioid peptides derived from plant proteins. *Current Pharmaceutical Design, 9*, 1325–1330.

Zioudrou, C., et al. (1979). Opioid peptides derived from food proteins: The exorphins. *Journal of Biological Chemistry, 254*, 2446–2449.

Chapter 4: Understanding and Testing for Celiac Disease

Abdulkarim, A., et al. (2002). Etiology of nonresponsive celiac disease: Results of a systematic response. *American Journal of Gastroenterology, 97*, 2016–2021.

Abrams, J., et al. (2004). Seronegative celiac disease: Increased prevalence with lesser degrees of villous atrophy. *Digestive Diseases and Sciences, 49*, 546–550.

Agardh, D., et al. (2002). Tissue transglutaminase autoantibodies and human leucocyte antigen in Down's syndrome patients with coeliac disease. *Acta Paediatrica, 91*, 34–38.

Aine, L., et al. (1990). Dental enamel defects in celiac disease. *Journal of Oral Pathology and Medicine, 19*, 241–245.

Alaedini, A., et al. (2002). Ganglioside reactive antibodies in the neuropathy associated with celiac disease. *Journal of Neuroimmunology, 127*, 145–148.

Askling, J., et al. (2002). Cancer incidence in a population-based cohort of individuals hospitalized with celiac disease or dermatitis herpetiformis. *Gastroenterology, 123*, 1428–1435.

Atkinson, M. A., & Eisenbarth, G. S. (2001). Type 1 diabetes: New perspectives on disease pathogenesis and treatment. *Lancet, 358*, 221–229.

Baker, A. L., & Rosenberg, I. H. (1978). Refractory sprue: recovery after removal of nongluten dietary proteins. *Annals of Internal Medicine, 89*, 505–508.

Bao, F., et al. (1999). One third of HLA DQ2 homozygous patients with type 1 diabetes express celiac disease-associated transglutaminase autoantibodies. *Journal of Autoimmunity, 13*, 143–148.

Basu, D., et al. (2000). Molecular basis for recognition of an arthritic peptide and a foreign epitope on distinct MHC molecules by a single TCR. *Journal of Immunology, 164*, 5788–5796.

Berger, E., et al. (1964). Demonstration of food antibodies in the feces or gastrointestinal tract in subjects allergic to cow's milk, in celiac disease and in non-allergic subjects. A. *Schweizerische medizinische Wochenschrift, 94*, 480–484.

Bevan, S., et al. (1999). Contribution of the MHC region to the familial risk of coeliac disease. *Journal of Medical Genetics, 36*, 687–690.

Bingley, P. J., et al. (2004). Undiagnosed coeliac disease at age seven: Population based prospective birth cohort study. *BMJ, 328*, 322–323.

Bonamico, M., et al. (2001). Radioimmunoassay to detect antitransglutaminase autoantibodies is the most sensitive and specific screening method for celiac disease. *American Journal of Gastroenterology, 96*, 1536–1540.

Bonamico, M., et al. (2002). Prevalence and clinical picture of celiac disease in Turner syndrome. *Journal of Clinical Endocrinology and Metabolism, 87*, 5495–5498.

Bonamico, M., et al. (2004a). Patchy villous atrophy of the duodenum in childhood celiac disease. *Journal of Pediatric Gastroenterology and Nutrition, 38,* 204–207.

Bonamico, M., et al. (2004b). Tissue transglutaminase autoantibody detection in human saliva: A powerful method for celiac disease screening. *Journal of Pediatrics, 144,* 632–636.

Bruce, S. E., et al. (1985). Human jejunal transglutaminase: Demonstration of activity, enzyme kinetics and substrate specificity with special relation to gliadin and coeliac disease. *Clinical Science (London), 68,* 573–579.

Bushara, K. O., et al. (2001). Gluten sensitivity in sporadic and hereditary cerebellar ataxia. *Annals of Neurology, 49,* 540–543.

Buzzetti, R., et al. (1998). Dissecting the genetics of type 1 diabetes: Relevance for familial clustering and differences in incidence. *Diabetes/ Metabolism Reviews, 14,* 111–128.

Carroccio, A., et al. (1993). Immunologic and absorptive tests in celiac disease: Can they replace intestinal biopsies? *Scandinavian Journal of Gastroenterology, 28,* 673–676.

Carroccio, A., et al. (2001). Guinea pig transglutaminase immunolinked assay does not predict celiac disease in patients with chronic liver disease. *Gut, 49,* 506–511.

Cataldo, F., et al. (1997). Celiac disease and selective immunoglobulin A deficiency. *Journal of Pediatrics, 131,* 306–308.

Cataldo, F., et al. (1998). Prevalence and clinical features of selective immunoglobulin A deficiency in coeliac disease: An Italian multicentre study. *Gut, 42,* 362–365.

Celiac Disease Center, Columbia University. (n.d.). *Serological and genetic testing.* Retrieved February 26, 2008, from http://www.celiac-diseasecenter.columbia.edu/C_Doctors/C05-Testing.htm

Cellier, C., et al. (1998). Abnormal intestinal intraepithelial lymphocytes in refractory sprue. *Gastroenterology, 114,* 471–481.

Cellier, C., et al. (2000). Refractory sprue, coeliac disease, and enteropathy-associated T-cell lymphoma. *Lancet, 256,* 203–208.

Chin, R. L., et al. (2004). Neurological complications of celiac disease. *Journal of Clinical Neuromuscular Disease, 5,* 129–137.

Ciacci, C., & Mazzacca, G. (1998). Unintentional gluten ingestion in celiac patients. *Gastroenterology, 115*, 243.

Clemente, M. G., et al. (2002). Antitissue transglutaminase antibodies outside celiac disease. *Journal of Pediatric Gastroenterology and Nutrition, 34*, 31–34.

Collin, P., et al. (2002). Endocrinological disorders and celiac disease. *Endocrine Reviews, 23*, 464–483.

Cooper, B. T. (1986). The delayed diagnosis of coeliac disease. *New Zealand Medical Journal, 99*, 543–545.

Corazza, G. R., et al. (1995). Celiac disease and alopecia areata: Report of a new association. *Gastroenterology, 109*, 1333–1337.

Corrao, G., et al. (2001). Mortality in patients with coeliac disease and their relatives: A cohort study. *Lancet, 358*, 356–361.

Curione, M., et al. (1999). Prevalence of coeliac disease in idiopathic dilated cardiomyopathy. *Lancet, 354*, 222–223.

Dahele, A., et al. (2001a). Anti-endomysial antibody negative celiac disease: Does additional serological testing help? *Digestive Diseases and Sciences, 46*, 214–221.

Dahele, A., et al. (2001b). Serum IgA tissue transglutaminase antibodies in coeliac disease and other gastrointestinal diseases. *Quarterly Journal of Medicine, 94*, 195–205.

Dalton, T. A., & Bennett, J. C. (1992). Autoimmune disease and the major histocompatibility complex: Therapeutic implications. *American Journal of Medicine, 92*, 183–188.

Dandalides, S. M., et al. (1989). Endoscopic small bowel mucosal biopsy: A controlled trial evaluating forceps size and biopsy location in the diagnosis of normal and abnormal mucosal architecture. *Gastrointestinal Endoscopy, 35*, 197–200.

Daum, S., et al. (1999). Increased expression of mRNA for matrix metalloproteinases-1 and -3 and tissue inhibitor of metalloproteinases-1 in intestinal biopsy specimens from patients with coeliac disease. *Gut, 44*, 17–25.

Davison, S. (2002). Coeliac disease and liver dysfunction. *Archives of Disease in Childhood, 87*, 293–296.

Dewar, D., et al. (2004). The pathogenesis of coeliac disease. *International Journal of Biochemistry and Cell Biology, 36,* 17–24.

Dickey, W., & Hughes, D. (2001). Disappointing sensitivity of endoscopic markers for villous atrophy in a high-risk population: Implications for celiac disease diagnosis during routine endoscopy. *American Journal of Gastroenterology, 96,* 2126–2128.

Dickey, W., & McConnell, J. B. (1996). How many hospital visits does it take before celiac sprue is diagnosed? *Journal of Clinical Gastroenterology, 23,* 21–23.

Dickey, W., et al. (2000). Reliance on serum endomysial antibody testing underestimates the true prevalence of coeliac disease by one fifth. *Scandinavian Journal of Gastroenterology, 35,* 181–183.

Dickey, W., et al. (2001). Sensitivity of serum tissue transglutaminase antibodies for endomysial antibody positive and negative coeliac disease. *Scandinavian Journal of Gastroenterology, 36,* 511–514.

Dieterich, W., et al. (1997). Identification of tissue transglutaminase as the autoantigen of celiac disease. *Nature Medicine, 3,* 797–801.

Dignass, A. U., & Podolsky, D. K. (1993). Cytokine modulation of intestinal epithelial cell restitution: Central role of transforming growth factor beta. *Gastroenterology, 105,* 1323–1332.

Di Leo, M., et al. (1993). Serum and salivary antiendomysium antibodies in the screening of coeliac disease. *Paninerva Medica, 41*(1), 68–71.

Dissanayake, A. S., et al. (1974). Jejunal mucosal recovery in coeliac disease in relation to the degree of adherence to a gluten-free diet. *Quarterly Journal of Medicine, 43,* 161–185.

Driscoll, H. K., et al. (1997). Vitamin A stimulation of insulin secretion: Effects on transglutaminase mRNA and activity using rat islets and insulin-secreting cells. *Pancreas, 15,* 69–77.

Esposito, C., et al. (2002). Anti tissue transglutaminase antibodies from coeliac patients inhibit transglutaminase activity both in vitro and in situ. *Gut, 51,* 177–181.

Esposito, C., et al. (2003). Expression and enzymatic activity of small intestinal tissue transglutaminase in celiac disease. *American Journal of Gastroenterology, 98,* 1813–1820.

Fasano, A., & Catassi, C. (2001). Current approaches to diagnosis and treatment of celiac disease: An evolving spectrum. *Gastroenterology, 120*, 636–651.

Fasano, A., et al. (2000). Zonulin, a newly discovered modulator of intestinal permeability, and its expression in coeliac disease. *Lancet, 355*, 1518–1519.

Fasano, A., et al. (2003). Prevalence of celiac disease in at-risk and not-at-risk groups in the United States: A large multicenter study. *Archives of Internal Medicine, 163*, 286–292.

Feighery, L., et al. (2003). Anti-transglutaminase antibodies and the serological diagnosis of coeliac disease. *British Journal of Biomedical Science, 60*, 14–18.

Fesus, L., & Piacentini, M. (2002). Transglutaminase 2: An enigmatic enzyme with diverse functions. *Trends in Biochemical Sciences, 27*, 534–539.

Fine, K. D., et al. (1997). The prevalence and causes of chronic diarrhea in patients with celiac sprue treated with a gluten-free diet. *Gastroenterology, 112*, 1830–1838.

Folk, J. E., & Chung, S. I. (1985). Transglutaminases. *Methods in Enzymology, 113*, 358–375.

Fourrier E. (1997). [Allergy to cow's milk]. *Allergie et immunologie, 29*(Spec. No.), 25–27.

Freeman, H. J. (2008). Pearls and pitfalls in the diagnosis of adult celiac disease. *Canadian Journal of Gastroenterology, 22*, 273–280.

Frustaci, A., et al. (2002). Celiac disease associated with autoimmune myocarditis. *Circulation, 105*, 2611–2618.

Fry, L. (2002). Dermatitis herpetiformis: Problems, progress and prospects. *European Journal of Dermatology, 12*, 523–531.

Gabrielli, M., et al. (2003). Association between migraine and celiac disease: Results from a preliminary case-control and therapeutic study. *American Journal of Gastroenterology, 98*, 625–629.

Gianfrani, C., et al. (2003). Celiac disease association with CD8 + T cell responses: Identification of a novel gliadin-derived HLA-A2-restricted epitope. *Journal of Immunology, 170*, 2719–2726.

Gillett, H. R., et al. (2000). Prevalence of IgA antibodies to endomysium and tissue transglutaminase in primary biliary cirrhosis. *Canadian Journal of Gastroenterology, 14,* 672–675.

Gookin, J. L., et al. (2002). Host responses to *Cryptosporidium* infection. *Journal of Veterinary Internal Medicine, 16*(1), 12–21.

Gomez, J. C., et al. (1998). Exocrine pancreatic insufficiency in celiac disease. *Gastroenterology, 114,* 621–623.

Gomis, R., et al. (1983). Transglutaminase activity in pancreatic islets. *Biochimica et Biophysica Acta, 760,* 384–388.

Green, P. H., & Jabri, B. (2003). Coeliac disease. *Lancet, 362,* 383–391.

Green, P. H., & Murray, J. A. (2003). Routine duodenal biopsies to exclude celiac disease? *Gastrointestinal Endoscopy, 58,* 92–95.

Green, P. H., et al. (2000). Significance of unsuspected celiac disease detected at endoscopy. *Gastrointestinal Endoscopy, 51,* 60–65.

Green, P. H., et al. (2003a). Risk of malignancy in patients with celiac disease. *American Journal of Medicine, 115*(3), 191–195.

Green, P. H., et al. (2003). Serologic tests for celiac disease. *Gastroenterology, 124,* 585–586.

Griffin, M., et al. (2002). Transglutaminases: Nature's biological glues. *Biochemical Journal, 368,* 377–396.

Haas, L., et al. (1993). Increased concentrations of fecal anti-gliadin IgA antibodies in untreated celiac disease. *Clinical Chemistry, 39,* 696–697.

Hadjivassiliou, M., et al. (1999). Idiopathic cerebellar ataxia associated with celiac disease: Lack of distinctive neurological features. *Journal of Neurology, Neurosurgery, and Psychiatry, 67,* 257.

Hadjivassiliou, M., et al. (2003). Dietary treatment of gluten ataxia. *Journal of Neurology, Neurosurgery, and Psychiatry, 74,* 1221–1224.

Halblaub, J. M., et al. (2004). Comparison of different salivary and fecal antibodies for the diagnosis of celiac disease. *Clinical Laboratory, 50,* 551–557.

Halttunen, T., et al. (1996). Fibroblasts and transforming growth factor beta induce organization and differentiation of T84 human epithelial cells. *Gastroenterology, 111,* 1252–1262.

Howell, M. D., et al. (1986). An HLA-D region restriction fragment length polymorphism associated with celiac disease. *Journal of Experimental Medicine, 164*, 333–338.

Hue, S., et al. (2004). A direct role for NKG2D/MICA interaction in villous atrophy during celiac disease. *Immunity, 21*, 367–377.

Hurlstone, D. P., & Sanders, D. S. (2003). High-magnification immersion chromoscopic duodenoscopy permits visualization of patchy atrophy in celiac disease: An opportunity to target biopsies of abnormal mucosa. *Gastrointestinal Endoscopy, 58*, 815–816.

Iltanen, S., et al. (1999). Celiac disease and markers of celiac disease latency in patients with primary Sjogren's syndrome. *American Journal of Gastroenterology, 94*, 1042–1046.

Jennings, J., et al. (2000). A new cause of "non-responsiveness" in celiac disease? *Postgraduate Medical Journal, 76*, 227–229.

Kaczmarski, M. (1995). The disaccharidase activity of jejunal mucosa in children with malabsorption syndrome caused by food intolerance. *Roczniki Akademii Medycznej im. Juliana Marchlewskiego w Bia?ymstoku, 40*, 504–511.

Kaplan, J. G., et al. (1988). Distal axonopathy associated with chronic gluten enteropathy: a treatable disorder. *Neurology, 38*, 642–645.

Kappler, M., et al. (2006). Detection of secretory IgA antibodies against gliadin and human tissue transglutaminase in stool to screen for coeliac disease in children: Validation study. *BMJ, 332*, 213–214.

Kaukinen, K., et al. (1999). No effect of gluten-free diet on the metabolic control of type 1 diabetes in patients with diabetes and celiac disease: Retrospective and controlled prospective survey. *Diabetes Care, 22*, 1747–1748.

Kemppainen, T., et al. (1999). Osteoporosis in adult patients with celiac disease. *Bone, 24*, 249–255.

Kokkonen, J., et al. (2001a). Cow's milk protein-sensitive enteropathy at school age. *Journal of Pediatrics, 139*, 797–803.

Kokkonen, J., et al. (2001b). Mucosal pathology of the foregut associated with food allergy and recurrent abdominal pains in children. *Acta Paediatrica, 90*(1), 16–21.

Koninckx, C. R., et al. (1984). IgA antigliadin antibodies in celiac and inflammatory bowel disease. *Journal of Pediatric Gastroenterology and Nutrition, 3,* 676–682.

Korponay-Szabo, I. R., et al. (2000). Tissue transglutaminase is the target in both rodent and primate tissues for celiac disease-specific autoantibodies. *Journal of Pediatric Gastroenterology and Nutrition, 31,* 520–527.

Korponay-Szabo, I. R., et al. (2003). Missing endomysial and reticulin binding of coeliac antibodies in transglutaminase 2 knockout tissues. *Gut, 52,* 199–204.

Lahteenoja, H., et al. (1999). Salivary antigliadin and antiendomysium antibodies in coeliac disease. *Scandinavian Journal of Immunology, 50,* 528–535.

Lai, T. S., et al. (1998). Regulation of human tissue transglutaminase function by magnesium-nucleotide complexes: Identification of distinct binding sites for Mg-GTP and Mg-ATP. *Journal of Biological Chemistry, 273,* 1776–1781.

Lampasona. V., et al. (1999). Antibodies to tissue transglutaminas C in type I diabetes. *Diabetologia, 42,* 1195–1198.

Lang, H. L., et al. (2002). A functional and structural basis for TCR cross-reactivity in multiple sclerosis. *Nature Immunology, 3,* 940–943.

Lankisch, P. G., et al. (1996). Diagnostic intervals for recognizing celiac disease. *Zeitschrift für Gastroenterologie, 34,* 473–477.

Lee, S. K., et al. (2003). Duodenal histology in patients with celiac disease after treatment with a gluten-free diet. *Gastrointestinal Endoscopy, 57,* 187–191.

Leon, F., et al. (2001). Anti-transglutaminase IgA ELISA: Clinical potential and drawbacks in celiac disease diagnosis. *Scandinavian Journal of Gastroenterology, 36,* 849–853.

Leong, R., et al. (2006, October). *Confocal laser endomicroscopy in the diagnosis of celiac disease.* Paper presented at the Australian Gastroenterology Week, Adelaide, South Australia, Australia.

Lepore, L., et al. (1993). Anti-alpha-gliadin antibodies are not predictive of celiac disease in juvenile chronic arthritis. *Acta Paediatrica, 82,* 569–573.

Lepore, L., et al. (1996). Prevalence of celiac disease in patients with juvenile chronic arthritis. *Journal of Pediatrics, 129,* 311–313.

Lo, W., et al. (2003). Changing presentation of adult celiac disease. *Digestive Diseases and Sciences, 48,* 395–398.

Lorand, L., & Conrad, S. M. (1984). Transglutaminases. *Molecular and Cellular Biochemistry, 58,* 9–35.

Luostarinen, L., et al. (2001). Association between coeliac disease, epilepsy and brain atrophy. *European Neurology, 46,* 187–191.

Luostarinen, L., et al. (2003). Neuromuscular and sensory disturbances in patients with well treated coeliac disease. *Journal of Neurology, Neurosurgery, and Psychiatry, 74,* 490–494.

Lundqvist, C., (1996). Intraepithelial lymphocytes in human gut have lytic potential and a cytokine profile that suggest T helper 1 and cytotoxic functions. *Journal of Immunology, 157,* 1926–1934.

Mainardi, E., et al. (2002). Thyroid-related autoantibodies and celiac disease: A role for a gluten-free diet? *Journal of Clinical Gastroenterology, 35,* 245–248.

Maki, M., et al. (2003). Prevalence of celiac disease among children in Finland. *New England Journal of Medicine, 348,* 2517–2524.

Marsh, M. N. (1992). Gluten, major histocompatibility complex, and the small intestine. A molecular and immunobiologic approach to the spectrum of gluten sensitivity ("celiac sprue"). *Gastroenterology, 102,* 330–354.

Marsh, M. N., & Crowe, P. T. (1995). Morphology of the mucosal lesion in gluten sensitivity. *Baillière's Clinical Gastroenterology, 9,* 273–293.

Meloni, G. F., et al. (1999). The prevalence of coeliac disease ininfertility. *Human Reproduction (Oxford, England), 14,* 2759–2761.

Meresse, B., et al. (2004). Coordinated induction by IL15 of a TCR-independent NKG2D signaling pathway converts CTL into lymphokine-activated killer cells in celiac disease. *Immunity, 21,* 357–366.

Molberg, O., et al. (2000). Role of tissue transglutaminase in celiac disease. *Journal of Pediatric Gastroenterology and Nutrition, 30,* 232–240.

Mori, M., et al. (1999). *Haemophilus influenzae* has a GM1 ganglioside-like structure and elicits Guillain-Barré syndrome. *Neurology, 52,* 1282–1284.

Muller, A. F., et al. (1996). Neurological complications of celiac disease: A rare but continuing problem. *American Journal of Gastroenterlogy, 91,* 1430–1435.

Murray, J. A., et al. (2003). Trends in the identification and clinical features of celiac disease in a North American community, 1950–2001. *Clinical Gastroenterology and Hepatology, 1,* 19–27.

National Institutes of Health Consensus Development Panel on Celiac Disease. (2004). Celiac disease. *Gastroenterology, 128*(4 Suppl. 1), S1–S9.

Nemes, Z., & Steinert, P. M. (1999). Bricks and mortar of the epidermal barrier. *Experimental and Molecular Medicine, 31,* 5–19.

Nichols, B. L., et al. (2000). Contribution of villous atrophy to reduced intestinal maltase in infants with malnutrition. *Journal of Pediatric Gastroenterology and Nutrition, 30,* 494–502.

Nunes, I., et al. (1997). Latent transforming growth factor-beta binding protein domains involved in activation and transglutaminase-dependent cross linking of latent transforming growth factor-beta. *Journal of Cell Biology, 136,* 1151–1163.

Oberhuber, G., et al. (1996). Evidence that intestinal intraepithelial lymphocytes are activated cytotoxic T cells in celiac disease but not in giardiasis. *American Journal of Pathology, 148,* 1351–1357.

O'Leary, C., et al. (2002). Coeliac disease and autoimmune Addison's disease: A clinical pitfall. *Quarterly Journal of Medicine, 95,* 79–82.

O'Mahony, S., et al. (1996). Management of patients with non-responsive coeliac disease. *Alimentary Pharmacology and Therapeutics, 10,* 671–680.

Oxentenko, A. S., et al. (2002). The insensitivity of endoscopic markers in celiac disease. *American Journal of Gastroenterology, 97,* 933–938.

Patey-Mariaud de Serre. N., et al. (2000). Distinction between celiac disease and refractory sprue: A simple immunohistochemical methods. *Histopathology, 37,* 70–77.

Pender, S. L., et al. (1997). A major role for matrix metalloproteinases in T cell injury in the gut. *Journal of Immunology, 158,* 1582–1590.

Peracchi, M., et al. (2002). Tissue transglutaminase antibodies in patients with end-stage heart failure. *American Journal of Gastroenterology, 97,* 2850–2854.

Picarelli, A., et al. (2002). Antiendomysial antibody detection in fecal supernatants: In vivo proof that small bowel mucosa is the site of antiendomysial antibody production. *American Journal of Gastroenterology, 97,* 95–98.

Polizzi, A., et al. (2000). Recurrent peripheral neuropathy in a girl with celiac disease. *Journal of Neurology, Neurosurgery, and Psychiatry, 68,* 104–105.

Porter, W. M., et al. (1999). Tissue transglutaminase antibodies in dermatitis herpetiformis. *Gastroenterology, 117,* 749–750.

Rampertab, S. D., et al. (2006). Trends in the presentation of celiac disease. *American Journal of Medicine, 119,* 335.e9–335.e14.

Ransford, R. A., et al. (2002). A controlled, prospective screening study of celiac disease presenting as iron deficiency anemia. *Journal of Clinical Gastroenterology, 35,* 228–233.

Reunala, T. L. (2001). Dermatitis herpetiformis. *Clinics in Dermatology, 19,* 728–736.

Rostami, K., et al. (1999a). The relationship between anti-endomysium antibodies and villous atrophy in coeliac disease using both monkey and human substrate. *European Journal of Gastroenterology and Hepatology, 11,* 439–442.

Rostami, K., et al. (1999b). Sensitivity of antiendomysium and antigliadin antibodies in untreated celiac disease: Disappointing in clinical practice. *American Journal of Gastroenterology, 94,* 888–894.

Rostami, K., et al. (2001). Coeliac disease and reproductive disorders: A neglected association. *European Journal of Obstetrics, Gynecology, and Reproductive Biology, 96*, 146–149.

Rostom, A., et al. (2004). *Celiac disease.* Evidence Report/Technology Assessment No. 104. Rockville, MD: Agency for Healthcare Research and Quality. (AHRQ publication no. 04-E029-2)

Ruoppolo, M., et al. (2003). Analysis of transglutaminase protein substrates by functional proteomics. *Protein Science, 12*, 1290–1297.

Ryan, B., & Kelleher, D. (2000). Refractory celiac disease. *Gastroenterology, 19*, 243–251.

Sanders, D. S., et al. (2001). Association of adult coeliac disease with irritable bowel syndrome: A case-control study in patients fulfilling ROME II criteria referred to secondary care. *Lancet, 358*, 1504–1508.

Sardy, M., et al. (1999). Recombinant human tissue transglutaminase ELISA for the diagnosis of gluten-sensitive enteropathy. *Clinical Chemistry, 45*, 2142–2149.

Sardy, M., et al. (2002). Epidermal transglutaminase (TGase 3) is the autoantigen of dermatitis herpetiformis. *Journal of Experimental Medicine, 195*, 747–757.

Sategna-Guidetti, C., et al. (1993). Serum IgA antiendomysium antibody titers as a marker of intestinal involvement and diet compliance in adult celiac sprue. *Journal of Clinical Gastroenterology, 17*, 123–127.

Sategna-Guidetti, C., et al. (1996). Reliability of immunologic markers of celiac sprue in the assessment of mucosal recovery after gluten withdrawal. *Journal of Clinical Gastroenterology, 23*, 101–104.

Savilahti, E. (2000). Food-induced malabsorption syndromes. *Journal of Pediatric Gastroenterology and Nutrition, 30*, S61–S66.

Sbarbati, A., et al. (2003). Gluten sensitivity and "normal" histology: Is the intestinal mucosa really normal? *Digestive and Liver Disease, 35*, 768–773.

Scott, B. B., & Losowsky, M. S. (1976). Patchiness and duodenal-jejunal variation of the mucosal abnormality in coeliac disease and dermatitis herpetiformis. *Gut, 17*, 984–992.

Shah, V. H., et al. (2000). All that scallops is not celiac disease. *Gastrointestinal Endoscopy, 51*, 717–720.

Shamir, R., et al. (2002). The use of a single serological marker underestimates the prevalence of celiac disease in Israel: A study of blood donors. *American Journal of Gastroenterology, 97,* 2589–2594.

Shan, L., et al. (2002). Structural basis for gluten intolerance in celiac sprue. *Science, 297,* 2275–2279.

Shill, H. A. (2003). Anti-ganglioside antibodies in idiopathic and hereditary cerebellar degeneration. *Neurology, 60,* 1672–1673.

Siegel, L. M., et al. (1997). Combined magnification endoscopy with chromoendoscopy in the evaluation of patients with suspected malabsorption. *Gastrointestinal Endoscopy, 46,* 226–230.

Sinclair, D., et al. (2006). Do we need to measure total serum IgA to exclude IgA deficiency in coeliac disease? *Journal of Clinical Pathology, 59,* 736–739.

Sjoberg, K., et al. (1997). Frequent occurrence of non-specific gliadin antibodies in chronic liver disease: Endomysial but not gliadin antibodies predict celiac disease in patients with chronic liver disease. *Scandinavian Journal of Gastroenterology, 32,* 1162–1167.

Sollid, L. M. (2000). Molecular basis of celiac disease. *Annual Review of Immunology, 18,* 53–81.

Sollid, L. M., et al. (1989). Evidence for a primary association of celiac disease to a particular HLA-DQ alpha/beta heterodimer. *Journal of Experimental Medicine, 169,* 345–350.

Song, D., et al. (2006). Confirmation and prevention of intestinal barrier dysfunction and bacterial translocation caused by methotrexate. *Digestive Diseases and Sciences, 51,* 1549–1556.

Spadaro, A., et al. (2002). [Anti-tissue transglutaminase antibodies in inflammatory and degenerative arthropathies]. *Reumatismo, 54,* 344–350.

Sulkanen, S., et al. (1998). Tissue transglutaminase autoantibody enzyme-linked immunosorbent assay in detecting celiac disease. *Gastroenterology, 115,* 1322–1328.

Talley, N. J., et al. (1994). Epidemiology of celiac sprue: A community-based study. *American Journal of Gastroenterology, 89,* 843–846.

Thompson, T. (2003). Oats and the gluten-free diet. *Journal of the American Dietetic Association, 103,* 376–379.

Thompson, T. (2004). Gluten contamination of commercial oat products in the United States. *New England Journal of Medicine, 351,* 2021–2022.

Tommasini, A., et al. (2004). Mass screening for coeliac disease using antihuman transglutaminase antibody assay. *Archives of Disease in Childhood, 89,* 512–515

Tursi, A., et al. (2001). Low prevalence of antigliadin and anti-endomysium antibodies in subclinical/silent celiac disease. *American Journal of Gastroenterology, 96,* 1507–1510.

Tursi, A., et al. (2003a). High prevalence of small intestinal bacterial overgrowth in celiac patients with persistence of gastrointestinal symptoms after gluten withdrawal. *American Journal of Gastroenterology, 98,* 839–843.

Tursi, A., et al. (2003b). Lack of usefulness of anti transglutaminase antibodies in assessing histologic recovery after gluten-free diet in celiac disease. *Journal of Clinical Gastroenterology, 37,* 387–391.

Tursi, A., et al. (2003c). Prevalence of antitissue transglutaminase antibodies in different degrees of intestinal damage in celiac disease. *Journal of Clinical Gastroenterology, 36,* 219–221.

Uibo, O., et al. (1993). Serum IgA anti-gliadin antibodies in an adult population sample: High prevalence without celiac disease. *Digestive Diseases and Sciences, 38,* 2034–2037.

Vecchi, M., et al. (2003). High rate of positive anti-tissue transglutaminase antibodies in chronic liver disease: Role of liver decompensation and of the antigen source. *Scandinavian Journal of Gastroenterology, 38,* 50–54.

Ventura, A., & Martelossi, S. (1997). Dental enamel defects and coeliac disease. *Archives of Disease in Childhood, 77,* 91.

Ventura, A., et al. (1999). Duration of exposure to gluten and risk for autoimmune disorders in patients with celiac disease. *Gastroenterology, 117,* 297–303.

Verkarre, V., et al. (2003). Refractory celiac sprue is a diffuse gastrointestinal disease. *Gut, 52,* 205–211.

Volta, U., et al. (1998). Frequency and significance of anti-gliadin and anti-endomysial antibodies in autoimmune hepatitis. *Digestive Diseases and Sciences, 43*, 2190–2195.

Volta, U., et al. (2001). High prevalence of celiac disease in Italian general population. *Digestive Diseases and Sciences, 46*, 1500–1505.

Walker-Smith, J. A., et al. (1990). Revised criteria for diagnosis of coeliac disease. Report of Working Group of European Society of Paediatric Gastroenterology and Nutrition. *Archives of Disease in Childhood, 65*, 909– 911.

Watters, E. (2006, November). DNA is not destiny. *Discover*, 32–37, 75.

Wong, R. C., et al. (2002). A comparison of 13 guinea pig and human anti-tissue transglutaminase antibody ELISA kits. *Journal of Clinical Pathology, 55*, 488–494.

Wucherpfennig, K. W., & Strominger, J. L. (1995). Molecular mimicry in T cell-mediated autoimmunity: Viral peptides activate human T cell clones specific for myelin basic protein. *Cell, 80*, 695–705.

Yuki, N., et al. (1993). A bacterium lipopolysaccharide that elicits Guillain-Barré syndrome has a GM1 ganglioside-like structure. *Journal of Experimental Medicine, 178*, 1771–1775.

Chapter 5: The Untold Story: Understanding and Testing for Non-Celiac Forms of Gluten Intolerance

Adams, S. (2007, February 12). *Celiac disease alternative medicine.* Retrieved February 26, 2008, from Celiac.com Web site: http://www.celiac.com/articles/1109/1/Celiac-Disease-Alternative-Medicine/Page1.html

Bogdanovic, J., et al. (2006). Airborne exposure to wheat allergens: Measurement by human immunoglobulin G4 and rabbit immunoglobulin G immunoassays. *Clinical and Experimental Allergy, 36*, 1168–1175.

Braly, J., & Hoggan, R. (2002). *Dangerous grains.* New York: Penguin-Putnam-Avery.

Calero, P., et al. (1996). IgA antigliadin antibodies as a screening method for nonovert celiac disease in children with insulin-dependent diabetes mellitus. *Journal of Pediatric Gastroenterology and Nutrition, 23,* 29–33.

Cooke, W., & Holmes, G. (1984). *Coeliac disease.* New York: Churchill Livingstone.

Fasano, A. (2003). Celiac disease — How to handle a clinical chameleon. *New England Journal of Medicine, 348,* 2568–2570.

Fasano, A., et al. (2003). Prevalence of celiac disease in at-risk and not-at-risk groups in the United States: A large multicenter study. *Archives of Internal Medicine,163*(3), 286–292.

Hadjivassiliou, M., et al. (1996). Does cryptic gluten sensitivity play a part in neurological illness? *Lancet, 347,* 369–371.

Hadjivassiliou, M., et al. (1998). Clinical, radiological, neurophysiological, and neuropathological characteristics of gluten ataxia. *Lancet, 352,* 1582–1585

Hadjivassiliou, M., et al. (1999). Gluten sensitivity: A many headed hydra. *British Medical Journal, 318,* 1710–1711.

Hadjivassiliou, M., et al. (2001). Headache and CNS white matter abnormalities associated with gluten sensitivity. *Neurology, 56,* 385–388.

Hadjivassiliou, M., et al. (2002a). The humoral response in the pathogenesis of gluten ataxia. *Neurology, 58,* 1221–1226.

Hadjivassiliou, M., et al. (2002b). Gluten sensitivity as a neurological illness. *Journal of Neurology, Neurosurgery, and Psychiatry, 72,* 560–563.

Hadjivassiliou, M., et al. (2003a). Dietary treatment of gluten ataxia. *Journal of Neurology, Neurosurgery, and Psychiatry, 74,* 1221–1224.

Hadjivassiliou, M., et al. (2003b). Gluten ataxia in perspective: Epidemiology, genetic susceptibility and clinical characteristics. *Brain, 126,* 685–691.

Hadjivassiliou, M., et al. (2004a). Gluten sensitivity masquerading as systemic lupus erythematosus. *Annals of the Rheumatic Diseases, 63,* 1501–1503.

Hadjivassiliou, M., et al. (2004b). The immunology of gluten sensitivity: Beyond the gut. *Trends in Immunology, 25,* 578–582.

Hadjivassiliou, M., et al. (2005). Multiple sclerosis and occult gluten sensitivity. *Neurology, 64,* 933–934.

Hadjivassiliou, M., et al. (2006). Autoantibody targeting of brain and intestinal transglutaminase in gluten ataxia. *Neurology, 66,* 373–377.

Hadjivassiliou, M., et al. (2006b). Neuropathy associated with gluten sensitivity. *Journal of Neurology, Neurosurgery, and Psychiatry, 72,* 1262–1266.

Hadjivassiliou, M., et al. (2007). Myopathy associated with gluten sensitivity. *Muscle and Nerve, 35,* 443–450.

Hur, G. Y., et al. (in press). Prevalence of work-related symptoms and serum-specific antibodies to wheat flour in exposed workers in the bakery industry [Electronic version]. *Respiratory Medicine.*

Kaukinen, K., et al. (1998). Small-bowel mucosal inflammation in reticulin or gliadin antibody-positive patients without villous atrophy. *Scandinavian Journal of Gastroenterology, 33,* 944–949.

Kaukinen, K., et al. (2001). Celiac disease without villous atrophy: Revision of criteria called for. *Digestive Diseases and Sciences, 46,* 879–887.

Kaukinen, K., et al. (2007). Latent coeliac disease or coeliac disease beyond villous atrophy? *Gut, 56,* 1339–1340.

Liu, E., et al. (2007). Natural history of antibodies to deamidated gliadin peptides and transglutaminase in early childhood celiac disease. *Journal of Pediatric Gastroenterology and Nutrition, 45,* 293–300.

Noh, G., et al. (2007). The clinical significance of food specific IgE/IgG4 in food specific atopic dermatitis. *Pediatric Allergy and Immunology, 18*(1), 63–70.

Wilkinson, I. D., et al. (2005). Cerebellar abnormalities on proton MR spectroscopy in gluten ataxia. *Journal of Neurology, Neurosurgery, and Psychiatry, 76,* 1011–1103.

Zars, S., et al. (2005). Food-specific IgG4 antibody-guided exclusion diet improves symptoms and rectal compliance in irritable bowel syndrome. *Scandinavian Journal of Gastroenterology, 40,* 800–807.

Zars, S., et al. (2005). Food-specific serum IgG4 and IgE titers to common food antigens in irritable bowel syndrome. *American Journal of Gastroenterology, 100,* 1550–1557.

Chapter 6: Conventional Wheat Allergies and Non-Gluten Wheat Reactions

Aas, M. H., & Halvorsen, R. (2005). [Diagnosing allergic reactions to ingested wheat in children]. *Tidsskr Nor Laegeforen, 125,* 3085–3087.

Battais, F., et al. (2005). Identification of IgE-binding epitopes on gliadins for patients with food allergy to wheat. *Allergy, 60,* 815–821.

Battais, F., et al. (2006). Wheat flour allergy: an entire diagnostic tool for complex allergy. *Allergie et immunologie, 38*(2), 59–61.

Bogdanovic, J., et al. (2006). Airborne exposure to wheat allergens: measurement by human immunoglobulin G4 and rabbit immunoglobulin G immunoassays. *Clinical and Experimental Allergy, 36,* 1168–1175.

Constantin, C., et al. (2005). Different profiles of wheat antigens are recognised by patients suffering from coeliac disease and IgE-mediated food allergy. *International Archives of Allergy and Immunology, 138*(3), 257–266.

Hur, G. Y., et al. (in press). Prevalence of work-related symptoms and serum-specific antibodies to wheat flour in exposed workers in the bakery industry [Electronic version]. *Respiratory Medicine.*

Kozai, H., et al. (2006). Wheat-dependent exercise-induced anaphylaxis in mice is caused by gliadin and glutenin treatments. *Immunology Letters, 102*(1), 83–90.

Lauriere, M., et al. (2006). Hydrolysed wheat proteins present in cosmetics can induce immediate hypersensitivities. *Contact Dermatitis, 54*(5), 283–289.

Matsuo, H., et al. (2005a). Molecular cloning, recombinant expression and IgE-binding epitope of omega-5 gliadin, a major allergen in wheat-dependent exercise-induced anaphylaxis. *FEBS Journal, 272,* 4431–4438.

Matsuo, H., et al. (2005b). Specific IgE determination to epitope peptides of omega-5 gliadin and high molecular weight glutenin subunit is a useful tool for diagnosis of wheat-dependent exercise-induced anaphylaxis. *Journal of Immunology, 175,* 8116–8122.

Noh, G., et al. (2007). The clinical significance of food specific IgE/IgG4 in food specific atopic dermatitis. *Pediatric Allergy and Immunology, 18*(1), 63–70.

Takagi, H., et al. (2005). A rice-based edible vaccine expressing multiple T cell epitopes induces oral tolerance for inhibition of Th2-mediated IgE responses. *Proceedings of the National Academy of Sciences of the United States of America, 102,* 17525–17530.

Chapter 7: Testing for Reactions to Wheat and Gluten

See Chapters 4, 5, and 6.

Chapter 8: Infants, Children, and Gluten Intolerance

Akobeng, A. K., & Heller, R. F. (2007). Assessing the population impact of low rates of breast feeding on asthma, coeliac disease and obesity: The use of a new statistical method. *Archives of Disease in Childhood, 92,* 471–472.

Carlsson, A., et al. (2006). Prevalence of celiac disease: Before and after a national change in feeding recommendations. *Scandinavian Journal of Gastroenterology, 41,* 553–558.

Chertok, I. R. (2007). The importance of exclusive breastfeeding in infants at risk for celiac disease. *American Journal of Maternal Child Nursing, 32*(1), 50–54.

Ciacci, C., et al. (1996). Celiac disease and pregnancy outcome. *American Journal of Gastroenterology, 91,* 718–722.

Greco, L., et al. (1985). The effect of early feeding on the onset of symptoms in celiac disease. *Journal of Pediatric Gastroenterology and Nutrition, 4,* 52–55.

Guandalini, S. (2007). The influence of gluten: Weaning recommendations for healthy children and children at risk for celiac disease. *Nestlé Nutrition Workshop Series: Paediatric Programme, 60*, 139–151.

Ivarsson, A., et al. (2002). Breast-feeding protects against celiac disease. *American Journal of Clinical Nutrition, 75*, 914–921.

Jarvinen, K. M., et al. (1999). Cow's milk challenge through human milk evokes immune responses in infants with cow's milk allergy. *Journal of Pediatrics, 135*, 506–512.

Luciano, A., et al. (2002). Catch-up growth and final height in celiac disease. *La Pediatria medica e chirurgica: Medical and surgical pediatrics, 24*(1), 9–12.

Schack-Nielsen, L., & Michaelsen, K. F. (2006). Breast feeding and future health. *Current Opinion in Clinical Nutrition and Metabolic Care, 9*, 289–296.

Turck, D. (2007). Later effects of breastfeeding practice: The evidence. *Nestlé Nutrition Workshop Series: Paediatric Programme, 60*, 31–42.

Chapter 9: Treating Gluten Intolerance and Wheat/Gluten Allergies

Ciacci, C., et al. (2005). Grown-up coeliac children: The effects of only a few years on a gluten-free diet in childhood. *Alimentary Pharmacology and Therapeutics, 21*, 421–429.

Vanderhoof, J. A., & Young, R. J. (2003). Role of probiotics in the management of patients with food allergy. *Annals of Allergy, Asthma, and Immunology, 90*(6 Suppl. 3), 99–103.

Chapter 10: Problems Common in Gluten Intolerance: Anemia, Iron Deficiency, Hypothyroidism, and Osteoporosis

See Chapters 3 and 4.

Chapter 11: Optimizing Good Health and the Healing Process

Fletcher, R. H., & Fairfield, K. M. (2002). Vitamins for chronic disease prevention in adults. *Journal of the American Medical Association, 287*, 3127–3129.

Chapter 12: Avoiding Gluten but Not Getting Better

Abdulkarim, A., et al. (2002). Etiology of nonresponsive celiac disease: Results of a systematic response. *American Journal of Gastroenterology, 97,* 2016–2021.

Adams, C. (n.d.). *Causes of non-responsive celiac disease — More than 50% continue to ingest gluten unknowingly.* Retrieved February 26, 2008, from Celiac.com Web site: http://www.celiac.com/articles/741/1/Causes-of-Non-responsive-Celiac-Disease — More-than-50-Continue-to-Ingest-Gluten-Unknowingly/Page1.html

Borowiec, A. M., & Fedorak, R. N. (2007). The role of probiotics in management of irritable bowel syndrome. *Current Gastroenterology Reports, 9,* 393–400.

Biagi, F., et al. (2004). A milligram of gluten a day keeps the mucosal recovery away: A case report. *Nutrition Reviews, 62,* 360–363.

Bousquet, P. J., et al. (2008). Assessing skin prick tests reliability in ECRHS-I. *Allergy, 63,* 341–346.

Chinoy, B., et al. (2005). Skin testing versus radioallergosorbent testing for indoor allergens. *Clinical and Molecular Allergy, 3*(1), 4.

Choi, I. S., et al. (2005). Sensitivity of the skin prick test and specificity of the serum-specific IgE test for airway responsiveness to house dust mites in asthma. *Journal of Asthma, 42*(3), 197–202.

Ciacci, C., & Mazzacca, G. (1998). Unintentional gluten ingestion in celiac patients. *Gastroenterology, 115,* 243.

Collado, M. C., et al. (2007). Role of commercial probiotic strains against human pathogen adhesion to intestinal mucus. *Letters in Applied Microbiology, 45,* 454–460.

Cranney, A., et al. (2007). The Canadian Celiac Health Survey. *Digestive Diseases and Sciences, 52,* 1087–1095.

Drisko, J., et al.(2006). Treating irritable bowel syndrome with a food elimination diet followed by food challenge and probiotics. *Journal of the American College of Nutrition, 25,* 514–522.

Grazioli, B., et al.(2006). *Giardia lamblia* infection in patients with irritable bowel syndrome and dyspepsia: A prospective study. *World Journal of Gastroenterology, 12,* 1941–1944.

Khan, W. I., & Collins, S. J. (2006). Gut motor function: Immunological control in enteric infection and inflammation. *Clinical and Experimental Immunology, 143*, 389–397.

Jennings, J., et al. (2000). A new cause of "non-responsiveness" in celiac disease? *Postgraduate Medical Journal, 76*, 227–229.

Kumar, R., et al. (2006). Relevance of serum IgE estimation in allergic bronchial asthma with special reference to food allergy. *Asian Pacific Journal of Allergy and Immunology, 24*(4), 191–199.

O'Mahony, S., et al. (1996). Management of patients with non-responsive coeliac disease. *Alimentary Pharmacology and Therapeutics, 10*, 671–680.

Ostblom, E., et al. (2008). Reported symptoms of food hypersensitivity and sensitization to common foods in 4-year-old children. *Acta Paediatrica, 97*, 85–90.

Ou-Yang, W. X., et al. (2008). [Application of food allergens specific IgG antibody detection in chronic diarrhea in children]. *Zhongguo Dang Dai Er Ke Za Zhi, 10*(1), 21–24.

Patey-Mariaud de Serre. N., et al. (2000). Distinction between celiac disease and refractory sprue: A simple immunohistochemical methods. *Histopathology, 37*, 70–77.

Rayan, H. Z., et al. (2007). Prevalence and clinical features of *Dientamoeba fragilis* infections in patients suspected to have intestinal parasitic infection. *Journal of the Egyptian Society of Parasitology, 37*, 599–608.

Ridout, S., et al. (2006). The diagnosis of Brazil nut allergy using history, skin prick tests, serum-specific immunoglobulin E and food challenges. *Clinical and Experimental Allergy, 36*, 226–232.

Ryan, B., & Kelleher, D. (2000). Refractory celiac disease. *Gastroenterology, 19*, 243–251.

Stark, D., et al. (2006). Irritable bowel syndrome: A review on the role of intestinal protozoa and the importance of their detection and diagnosis. *International Journal for Parasitology, 37*(1), 11–20.

Tursi, A., et al. (2003a). High prevalence of small intestinal bacterial overgrowth in celiac patients with persistence of gastrointestinal symptoms after gluten withdrawal. *American Journal of Gastroenterology, 98,* 839–843.

Tursi, A., et al. (2006). Endoscopic and histological findings in the duodenum of adults with celiac disease before and after changing to a gluten-free diet: A 2-year prospective study. *Endoscopy, 38,* 702–707.

Uz, E., et al.(2007). Risk factors for irritable bowel syndrome in Turkish population: Role of food allergy [Abstract]. *Journal of Clinical Gastroenterology, 41,* 380–383.

Verkarre, V., et al. (2003). Refractory celiac sprue is a diffuse gastrointestinal disease. *Gut, 52,* 205–211.

Wahnschaffe, U., et al. (2007). Predictors of clinical response to gluten-free diet in patients diagnosed with diarrhea-predominant irritable bowel syndrome. *Clinical Gastroenterology and Hepatology, 5,* 844–850.

Wang, de Y., et al. (2007). Potential non-immunoglobulin E-mediated food allergies: Comparison of open challenge and double-blind placebo-controlled food challenge. *Otolaryngology — Head and Neck Surgery, 137,* 803–809.

Whorwell, P. J., et al. (2006). Efficacy of an encapsulated probiotic Bifidobacterium infantis 35624 in women with irritable bowel syndrome [Abstract]. *American Journal of Gastroenterology, 101,* 1581–1590.

Wood, J. D. (2006). Histamine, mast cells, and the enteric nervous system in the irritable bowel syndrome, enteritis, and food allergies. *Gut, 55,* 445–447.

Yang, C. M., & Li, Y. Q. (2007). [The therapeutic effects of eliminating allergic foods according to food-specific IgG antibodies in irritable bowel syndrome]. *Zhonghua Nei Ke Za Zhi, 46,* 641–643.

Zuo, X. L., et al. (2007). Alterations of food antigen-specific serum immunoglobulins G and E antibodies in patients with irritable bowel syndrome and functional dyspepsia. *Clinical and Experimental Allergy, 37,* 823–830.

Index

About the Author

Dr. Stephen Wangen is a state licensed and board certified physician. He received his doctoral degree in naturopathic medicine from internationally renowned Bastyr University. He practices in Seattle, Washington, in the Nordstrom Medical Tower at Swedish Medical Center and specializes in digestive disorders and food allergies. He is a founder of the Irritable Bowel Syndrome Treatment Center (www.IBSTreatmentCenter.com), where he serves as the medical director, and is on the board of the Gluten Intolerance Group of North America (www.gluten.net), a non-profit organization dedicated to providing support to people with all types of gluten intolerance.

In addition to the IBS Treatment Center, he has founded the Center for Food Allergies (www.CenterforFoodAllergies.com). His extensive research into the relationship between food allergies and health has led to groundbreaking work on many conditions. He continues to investigate these issues as the research director of the Innate Health Foundation (www.InnateHealthFoundation.org), a non-profit agency dedicated to the advancement of health and healthcare. His enthusiasm for healthcare is the result of a lifelong interest in human potential.

Media

Dr. Wangen is available for interviews and public speaking. For more information please contact Thomas Mercer, Public Relations Manager, at tmercer@IBSTreatmentCenter.com or by phone at 206-264-1111 or 1-888-546-6283.

Food Industry

Dr. Wangen is available for consultation on food products regarding food allergies and intolerances. For more information please contact Thomas Mercer, Public Relations Manager, at tmercer@ IBSTreatmentCenter.com or by phone at 206-264-1111 or 1-888-546-6283.

Researchers

Dr. Wangen is available for consultation for those designing studies or evaluating the results of research on gluten intolerance and food allergies. For more information please contact Dr. Wangen at info@IBSTreatmentCenter.com or by phone at 206-264-1111 or 1-888-546-6283.

Also by
Dr. Stephen Wangen

The Irritable Bowel Syndrome Solution:
How It's Cured At the IBS Treatment Center.

The authoritative resource
on IBS. Available at
www.IBSTreatmentCenter.com.

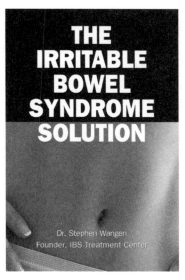

Email Newsletters

If you found this book interesting, you may like to get regular
health updates from the author and the Innate Health Group. Just
send an email telling us you'd like to subscribe to our newsletter
to info@IBSTreatmentCenter.com and we'll send you our free
monthly email newsletters.

Author's Blog

You can also read Dr. Wangen's blog, found at www.IBSTreat-
mentCenter.com.
His blog is available as an RSS feed.

Order
Form

Healthier Without Wheat $19.95
The Irritable Bowel Syndrome Solution $14.95

Online   www.IBSTreatmentCenter.com

By Phone   IBS Treatment Center, 206-264-1111,
toll free 1-888-546-6283

By Mail   Innate Health Publishing, 1229 Madison St.,
Suite 1220, Seattle, WA, 98104.

Name_____

Address _____

City _____State _____ Zip _____

Telephone _____

Email _____

Please Send Me:

Healthier Without Wheat   _____ copies @ $19.95 _____

The Irritable Bowel Syndrome Solution   _____ copies @ $14.95 _____

Tax   (WA residents only, add 8.9% tax,   _____
for each book shipped within the state of Washington.)

Shipping   (U.S. shipping: $4.00 for the first book,   _____
$2.00 for each additional book. International shipping:
$9.00 for the first book, $5.00 for each additional book.)

Total $ _____

Payment   ❏ Check   ❏ Visa   ❏ MasterCard

Credit card number _____

Name on card _____

Exp. date _____   Signature _____